Managing Pres Prevention

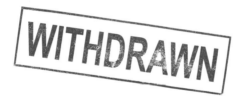

Other titles in the Key Management Skills in Nursing series

Key Management Skills in Nursing Series

Editors: R A Brown and G Castledine

Managing Pressure Sore Prevention

by
Carol Dealey

Quay
Books

Quay Books
Division of Mark Allen Publishing Limited
Jesses Farm, Snow Hill, Dinton, Nr Salisbury, Wilts, SP3 5HN

© Mark Allen Publishing Ltd, 1997

British Library Cataloguing-in-Publication Data

A catalogue record for this book is available from the British
Library
ISBN 1-85642-105 8

Printed in the UK by Biddles Limited, Guildford, Surrey

Contents

Acknowledgements

To my husband for his constant support and to Anne for reviewing my work.

Chapter 1
The politicisation of pressure sores

Introduction

Pressure sores are an unpleasant complication of illness or disability. They can be defined as ulceration of the skin following disruption of the blood supply due to pressure, friction or shear or any combination of these (Dealey, 1994a). Pressure sores are also known as pressure ulcers, decubitus ulcers or bedsores. The earliest known pressure sore that was found on the mummy of an ancient Egyptian priestess. The mummy was noted to have pieces of leather over the sores on the sacrum and buttocks (Rowling, 1961).

Historical background

Until recently, pressure sores were considered to be a nursing problem and of little interest to other healthcare professionals. Today, they are deemed to be an indicator of the quality of care provided by a hospital or unit and have been the subject of debate in the House of Lords (*Hansard*, 1993). An all-party parliamentary group on the subject of skin care has been set up. To understand how this change has come about, a historical perspective is needed.

Any investigator into nursing history tends to start with

Florence Nightingale. She had an opinion on pressure sores as she did on most other topics. She maintained that pressure sores could be prevented by good nursing care (Nightingale, 1961). Over time this view became reversed: rather than believing that good nursing prevented pressure sores, bad nursing was considered to cause them. As a result, the development of pressure sores in patients produced great feelings of guilt among nurses. Hibbs (1988) described pressure sores as a 'hidden epidemic beneath the bed-clothes.'

Dr Jean-Martin Charcot (1825–1893) was one of the first neurologists and had great influence in his day. He suggested that pressure sores in patients with spinal injuries were a consequence of the release of neurogenic trophic factors and that doctors could do nothing about them (Charcot, 1879). Variations on Charcot's theory appeared in a nursing textbook in 1946. Here pressure sores were also described as an inevitable consequence of spinal injury. Pearce (1946) suggested that 'a trophic ulcer is one that occurs because the nutritional nerves are affected...' Bedsores, however, were seen as rather different. There was some understanding that pressure might be a factor and the 'back round' was a major part of the nursing day. At regular intervals, nurses would treat the pressure areas of bedfast patients by washing and massaging them vigorously with soap and water. The pressure areas were then anointed with a variety of substances such as powder, oil and spirit or cream. This practice continued up to the 1970s in some areas.

The concept that doctors could do nothing about pressure sores persisted for many years. Medical textbooks published in the middle of this century described pressure sores as a nursing problem and, as a result, did not discuss their aetiology and management.

It was only in the 1980s that pressure sores started to attract attention from a wider audience. The Tissue Viability Society was established in 1980. The driving force of the society was and is a multidisciplinary approach. It has helped to establish the concept of tissue viability and the care and prevention of wounds of all types. Some of the medical members who were interested in pressure sores were able to influence a report on disability by the Royal College of Physicians (1986) entitled *Disability in 1986 and Beyond*. This was the first major policy document to include pressure sores. The document made a number of recommendations, some of which indicated a change in attitude by the physicians. The report suggested that there should be a district pressure sore service run by a senior nurse and a designated member of the medical staff. There should also be access to a plastic surgeon when necessary. It was suggested that there should be a written policy for the prevention and management of pressure sores. Although this report did not herald a new interest in pressure sores among senior doctors and hospital managers, it can be seen as a straw in the wind.

Bliss (1990), in an editorial in *The Lancet*, suggested that pressure sores should not be seen as a failure of nursing care but as a failure of a doctor to recognise the vulnerability of acutely ill or newly paralysed patients. There has been a gradual increase in the number of similar papers in medical journals, although there is still not the same degree of interest as in the nursing journals.

Sadly, the need to include the prevention and management of pressure sores in undergraduate medical training is still not considered of great importance. In a survey of UK medical schools, Bennett (1992) found that the time allocated to teaching the care and prevention of chronic wounds ranged from 0 to 36 hours, with an average of 6 hours. Bennett suggested that until pressure sores are included in those subjects on which medical students are examined, they are likely to be of little interest to them.

The cost of pressure sores

As the discussion of pressure sores has increased so, too has awareness of the costs they incur. Various estimates of the cost to the health service have been made. Fernie (1973) estimated that there were 60 000 pressure sores each year and calculated the cost of treatment to be £1000 per sore. Thus, pressure sores cost £60 million each year to treat. These figures should be viewed with caution, however, as they were derived from guesswork rather than known facts. Furthermore, some of the later authors have simply taken Fernie's figures and adjusted them according to inflation. Scales *et al* (1982) suggested that the total cost was more than £150 million per annum. Waterlow (1988) suggested that it cost about £300 million each year to treat pressure sores.

Hibbs (1988) found the cost of treating one patient with a deep pressure sore to be £25 905.58. She went further and calculated the opportunity costs, ie. what other use could have been made of the money. The patient referred to in the study was in an orthopaedic bed for 180 days, during which time 16 patients could have had a hip or knee replacement for the same cost.

The Nursing Practice Research Unit (1992) studied one district general hospital to determine the annual cost of the management and prevention of pressure sores. They suggested that the total cost was £408 311.05, of which £83 355.78 was incurred by the two orthopaedic wards. Preston (1991) considered the cost of pressure sore management in the community. He implied that upwards of £250 000 was spent each year in treating pressure sores in a community unit. Clough (1994) calculated that it cost £150 per patient to prevent pressure sores within an intensive care unit but £320 to treat them.

The cost of treatment may not be the only cost incurred by a hospital. There is increasing use of litigation by patients and/or their relatives. In 1987, a patient was awarded £98 000 damages following the development of a hospital-acquired pressure sore (Silver, 1987). Other litigants have since been successful, but many have accepted out-of-court settlements and the damages, therefore, are unknown.

As reference to the cost of pressure sores was increasingly made in the literature, the Department of Health commissioned a report into the cost of pressure sores (Touche Ross & Co, 1993). The authors of this report estimated the costs for a 600-bed district general hospital and described them in terms of low cost and high cost prevention or treatment. While low cost prevention was considered to cost the same as low cost treatment (£644 000), high cost prevention (£2 710 000) cost much more than high cost treatments (£1 153 000). However, there are a number of flaws in these estimates. The costings for prevention include the cost of staff education and employing a tissue viability nurse specialist, but assume that neither need to be included in the costs of treatment. They also consider that the treatment of pressure sores takes less staff time than prevention, whereas the converse is likely to be true.

The epidemiology of pressure sores

Pressure sores incur costs which can seem to be out of all proportion to their numbers. Several studies have been undertaken to identify patients with pressure sores in a variety of healthcare settings. It is difficult to compare these surveys as they have different methodologies and exclusions. They may be either prevalence or incidence surveys and it is important to be aware of the difference. There often seems to be confusion between the two and the terms are sometimes used interchangeably, despite having different meanings.

- **Prevalence** is the number of persons with a specific disease or condition as a proportion of a given population, measured at a specific point in time or over a specific period of time. Point prevalence is most frequently measured..

- **Incidence** is the number of persons developing a specific disease or condition as a proportion of the given population, measured over a period of time.

(Dealey, 1993)

Although a number of pressure sore prevalence surveys have been published, only the larger surveys from 1980 onwards are considered here. Ek and Bowman (1982) published the findings of a survey of public health service areas in Sweden which showed a 4% prevalence of pressure sores. For a considerable time this was considered to be the 'gold standard' which everyone should be striving to achieve. David *et al* (1983) surveyed 20 health districts within four health regions, excluding paediatrics, maternity, mental subnormality and acute psychiatry and found a prevalence of 6.7%. Nyquist and Hawthorn (1987) using the same methodology in a survey of an area health authority, found a prevalence of 5.78%. Girvin and Griffiths Jones (1989) surveyed 1010 patients and found a prevalence of 10.2% — higher than some of the earlier surveys. Clark and Cullum (1992) obtained similar results in their study, with a prevalence of 10.3%. In a survey of 3213 patients in a number of hospitals across the UK, O'Dea (1993) found a prevalence of 18.6%, which was considerably higher than that found in other surveys on this scale.

It is interesting to speculate why the prevalence rates have increased and whether the increase is real or apparent. It has been suggested that with increased understanding of pressure sore aetiology and removal of blame, nursing staff feel able to report more honestly than before, thus increasing the numbers of reported sores. Another possibility is that there are more patients with pressure sores. Of course, this is not a uniform picture. Dealey (1994b) compared two surveys, one carried out in 1989 and the other in 1993. She found a small reduction in pressure sore prevalence from 8.77% in 1989 to 7.9% in 1993, but the difference was not statistically significant.

While prevalence surveys can provide useful baseline information, incidence surveys are considered to be a more accurate measurement of pressure sore development. Prevalence surveys provide only a snapshot of the situation and do not differentiate between those admitted to a hospital or unit with a pressure sore, and those developing sores after admission. The measurement of incidence gives a truer picture because it is taken over time and identifies those patients developing sores while in a particular place of care.

One of the best-known incidence studies is that by Versluysen (1986) who studied 100 consecutive patients over 70 years of age admitted to a teaching hospital with fractured neck of femur. The incidence of pressure sores was a staggering 66% over an 18 month period. Gebhardt (1992) looked at 74 patients aged 62–99 years with the same diagnosis and found an annual incidence of 43%. In a study of a wider range of patients in a single NHS trust hospital, Clark and Watts (1994) found an annual incidence of 4.03% ranging from 1.8% in surgical wards to 10.3% in orthopaedic wards. This emphasises the differences that can occur between different patient groups.

Policy documents and pressure sores

During the last few years, a number of policy documents have been published which reflect the increased interest in pressure sores. In 1991 the Audit Commission Review entitled *The Virtue of Patients: Making the Best Use of Ward Nursing Resources* suggested that the incidence of pressure sores could be used as a marker of quality standards within a hospital. The following year *The Health of the Nation* document (Department of Health, 1992) recommended that one of the health targets should be an annual reduction in the incidence of pressure sores. It suggested that a reduction of 5–10% was reasonable.

The US government has also shown an interest in pressure sores. This has led to the Agency for Health Care Policy and Research (part of the US Department of Health and Human Sciences) developing a series of clinical practice guidelines relating to pressure sores (Panel for the Prediction and Prevention of Pressure Ulcers, 1992). These guidelines have been published in the form of monographs for both clinicians and patients and carers. They are available free of charge and copyright has been waived so that they can be adapted for local use.

In 1993, the Department of Health further indicated the importance of pressure sore prevention by publishing a document entitled *Pressure Sores: A Key Quality Indicator* (Department of Health, 1993). The purpose of the document was to provide information and guidance to both purchasers and providers within the NHS. Although it contains useful information for those with little understanding of the seriousness of pressure sores, it is rather superficial in content. Perhaps the most important aspect of the document is that it came to the attention of senior managers who would normally have little or no interest in the topic.

The NHS Executive has supported an initiative to develop a number of clinical guidelines at national level. Pressure sores were one of the topics deemed suitable. Clinical guidelines can be defined as:

> *'Standardised specifications for care developed by a formal process that incorporates the best scientific evidence of effectiveness with expert opinion.'*
>
> (Leape, 1990)

Their purpose is to assist practitioners in making decisions about care. The pressure sore guidelines were released in 1995. They form the basis of a number of the topics relating to pressure sore prevention and management discussed in this book.

The politics of pressure sores

In June 1993, pressure sores were the subject of debate in the House of Lords. In this debate, *The Health of the Nation* targets were discussed along with the need for specialist nurses who were knowledgeable in the use of pressure-relieving equipment. It could be considered that pressure sores had 'arrived' politically.

Thus, in a relatively short time, pressure sores have moved high up the political agenda. This is pleasing to those involved in the prevention and management of pressure sores. However, it also means that those with less knowledge of the topic are making political statements. There is anecdotal evidence of several chairmen of regional health authorities stating that they expect to achieve 0% pressure sore incidence in their regions. While this is a rather unrealistic target, it should be recognised that a few years ago pressure sores would have been of little interest to such senior figures. Therefore, while pressure sores are considered to be so important, nurses must get political and use the opportunity to improve patient care. This can be achieved by obtaining support for the development of local prevention strategies and educational programmes for the healthcare team.

Key points

1. Pressure sores can no longer be considered solely a nursing problem

2. While the total cost of pressure sores is uncertain, the costs in terms of personal suffering and hospital

costs are considerable

3. Measuring pressure sore prevalence provides useful baseline data

4. Pressure sore incidence provides a more accurate measure of quality of care provided by a hospital unit

5. Pressure sores have become a political issue; nurses can make use of this to improve patient care

References

Audit Commission Review (1991) *The Virtue of Patients: Making the Best of Ward Nursing Resources.* The Audit Commission for Local Authorities and the National Health Service in England and Wales, London

Bennett G (1992) Medical undergraduate teaching in chronic wound care (a survey). *J Tissue Viabil* **2**(2): 50–1

Bliss M (1990) Preventing pressure sores. (Editorial). *Lancet* **335**: 1311–12

Charcot JM (1879) *Lectures on the Disease of the Nervous System 'La Saltpetiere'.* Translated from the 2nd edn by Sigerson G, Henry C. Lea, Philadelphia

Clark M, Cullum N (1992) Matching patient need for pressure sore prevention with the supply of pressure redistributing mattresses. *J Adv Nurs* **17**: 310–16

Clark M, Watts S (1994) The incidence of pressure sores within a National Health Service trust hospital during 1991. *J Adv Nurs* **20**: 33–6

Clough NP (1994) The cost of pressure area management in an intensive care unit. *J Wound Care* **3**(1): 33–5

David JA, Chapman RG, Chapman EJ, Lockett B (1983) *An Investigation of the Current Methods Used in Nursing for the Care of Patients with Established Pressure Sores.* Nursing Practice Research Unit, Norwick Park, Middlesex

Dealey C (1993) Pressure sores: the result of bad nursing?

(Editorial). *Br J Nurs* **1**(15): 748

Dealey C (1994a) *The Care of Wounds*. Blackwell Scientific Publications, Oxford

Dealey C (1994b) Monitoring the pressure sore problem in a teaching hospital. *J Adv Nurs* **20**: 652–9

Department of Health (1992) *The Health of the Nation*. HMSO, London

Department of Health (1993) *Pressure Sores: A Key Quality Indicator*. Department of Health, London

Ek A-C, Bowman G (1982) A descriptive study of pressure sores: the prevalence of pressure sores and the characteristics of patients. *J Adv Nurs* **7**: 51–7

Fernie GR (1973) Biomechanical aspects of the aetiology of decubitus ulcers on human patients. PhD Thesis, University of Strathclyde, Glasgow

Gebhardt K (1992) Preventing pressure sores in orthopaedics. *Nurs Stand* **6**(23): 3–5

Girvin J, Griffiths Jones A (1989) Towards prevention, Journal of Wound Care Nursing. *Nurs Times* **85**(12): 64–6

Hansard (1993) Report on Parliamentary Proceedings, June 8

Hibbs P (1988) *Pressure Area Care for the City and Hackney Health Authority*. City and Hackney Health Authority, London

Leape L (1990) Practice guidelines: an overview. *Qual Rev Bull* **16**: 42–9

Nightingale F (1961) *Notes on Nursing*. Appleton Century, New York

Nursing Practice Research Unit (1992) *The Financial Costs of Pressure Sores to the National Health Service*. University of Surrey, Guildford

Nyquist R, Hawthorn PJ (1987) The prevalence of pressure sores within an area health authority. *J Adv Nurs* **12**: 183–7

O'Dea K (1993) Prevalence of pressure damage in hospital patients in the UK. *J Wound Care* **2**(4): 221–5

Panel for the Prediction and Prevention of Pressure Ulcers in Adults (1992) *Pressure Ulcers in Adults: Prediction and*

Prevention. AHCPR Publication, US Department of Health and Human Services, Rockville, Maryland

Pearce ECA (1946) *A General Textbook of Nursing*. Faber & Faber, London

Preston K (1991) Counting the cost of pressure sores. *Community Outlook* **1**(9): 19–24

Rowling JT (1961) Pathological changes in mummies. *Proc R Soc Med (London)* **54**: 409–15

Royal College of Physicians (1986) Disability in 1986 and beyond. *J R Coll Physicians Lond* **20**(3): 160–94

Scales JT, Lowthian PT, Poole AG, Ludman WR (1982) Vaperm Patient-Support System: a new general purpose hospital mattress. *Lancet* **ii**: 1150–2

Silver J (1987) Letter. *Care Sci Pract* **5**: 30

Touche Ross & Co (1993) *The Costs of Pressure Sores*. Department of Health, London

Versluysen M (1986) How elderly patients with femoral fracture develop pressure sores in hospital. *Br Med J* **292**: 1311–13

Waterlow J (1988) Prevention is cheaper than cure. *Nurs Times* **84**(25): 69–70

Chapter 2
The causes of pressure sores

Introduction

Before any pressure sore prevention programme can be established it is essential that the nurse understands the causes of pressure sores. A number of factors are involved: these can be divided into extrinsic, intrinsic and external factors. Each group will be considered in turn.

Extrinsic factors

The three extrinsic factors involved in pressure damage are pressure, friction and shear. The most important factor in pressure sore development is pressure, in particular pressure over a bony prominence or pressure area (*Figure 2.1*). External pressure over the tissues causes compression and distortion. If the pressure is sufficiently higher than capillary closing pressure it will result in occlusion of the blood vessels. Prolonged pressure can potentially lead to ischaemia and cell death.

Several aspects of this statement require further discussion. Landis (1931) was the first to attempt to measure the pressure within the capillaries. He used young, healthy students for his experiments. His results showed an average pressure of 32 mmHg at the arteriolar end of the capillary bed and 12 mmHg at the venule end. Thus, capillary closing

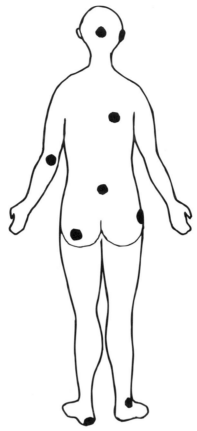

Figure 2.1: The bony prominences

pressure is generally quoted as being 32 mmHg. However, this can be misleading as capillary closing pressure may be quite different in an older person. Bridel (1993) suggested that the collagen content of the skin must also be considered, as collagen acts as a buffer to external pressure and provides some protection for the blood vessels.

Not everyone who sits or lies on a hard surface that exerts a high pressures develops a pressure sore. This is because tissue ischaemia results in localised discomfort or pain, causing the individual to move to another position. The relief of pressure is normally followed by reactive hyperaemia.

This is a temporary dilatation of the capillaries which brings oxygen to the area and removes the accumulated carbon dioxide and other waste products. It is characterised by a reddened area on the skin surface.

The extent of the damage caused by pressure is a function of the degree of localised pressure and its duration. In other words, damage can result from high pressures over short periods or from lower pressures over longer periods. However, there is no clear-cut evidence that defines the pressure/time ratio at which pressure damage occurs. Bridel (1993) suggests that once the critical values for pressure and time have been reached, tissue damage will proceed at a similar rate regardless of the degree of pressure being applied.

Distortion or tissue deformation may also be more important than has previously been recognised. Gebhardt (1995) argues that pressure is rarely applied uniformly and there is, therefore, a degree of tissue deformation which creates shear forces that can damage the blood vessels. Shearing also occurs if the patient slides down in the bed or chair. The skeleton moves but the skin stays still. The shear forces cause small blood vessels to tear, leading to disruption of the local blood supply which may be followed by ischaemia and cell death.

The other extrinsic factor to consider is friction. Friction can be described as the force generated when two surfaces move across one another (Krouskop, 1978). It can result in superficial damage, such as stripping of the epidermis. It is exacerbated by the presence of moisture.

Intrinsic factors

It is well recognised that it is the combination of a number of intrinsic factors that predisposes an individual to pressure sore development. If any extrinsic factor occurs, tissue damage will result.

A number of studies have shown that increasing age is a significant intrinsic factor in pressure sore development. David *et al* (1983) found that 85% of patients with pressure sores were over 65 years of age. In a comparison of two prevalence surveys in a teaching hospital, Dealey (1994) found that 62.9% of patients with pressure sores in one survey and 46.4% of patients in the second survey were over 65 years of age. This vulnerability can be explained by the fact that neurological and cardiovascular diseases increase with age. The skin also undergoes a number of changes with age, becoming thinner and less elastic and resilient. This is in part because the collagen content of the dermis reduces with age (Hall *et al*, 1981).

Schubert (1992) suggests that a low systolic blood pressure may also be a factor in pressure sore development in the elderly. He studied a group of elderly patients of whom 30 had pressure sores and 100 did not. He found that the patients with pressure sores had a significantly lower systolic blood pressure compared with the control group. An impaired reactive hyperaemia response was also found to correspond with a low systolic blood pressure.

Another factor considered to be of importance is reduced mobility. A number of prevalence surveys have identified reduced mobility as a factor in pressure sore development (David *et al*, 1983; Dealey, 1994). The inability to move easily or freely means that the individual is not able to relieve pressure over the pressure areas. If this person is immobile there is also the potential for sliding down in the bed or chair, causing shear or friction. Reduced mobility may be due to a number of factors. It may be short term, as in a patient undergoing major surgery or suffering traumatic injury. Versluysen (1986) studied 100 patients aged 70–94 years who had suffered a fractured neck of femur. She found a pressure sore incidence of 66%. Patients with chronic illness or disability may also have reduced mobility. Patients with rheumatoid arthritis are one example: not only are they likely to have poor mobility but also the use of steroids reduces the collagen content of the dermis, resulting in thinning skin which tears easily (Hall *et al*, 1974). Changing position to relieve pressure depends on the individual's ability to move and an awareness of the need to do so. Neurological deficit may mean that there is a loss of sensation and that the person is insensitive to pain. Gebhardt (1995) argues that loss of sensation is of greater significance than reduced mobility. The immobile patient with full sensation can ask to be moved when uncomfortable, whereas the insensate patient will not be stimulated to move and may accept prolonged pressure, resulting in pressure sore development. This can affect some patients who have no mobility problems, such as diabetic patients with peripheral neuropathy, as well as those with mobility problems, such as stroke patients or those with spinal injury.

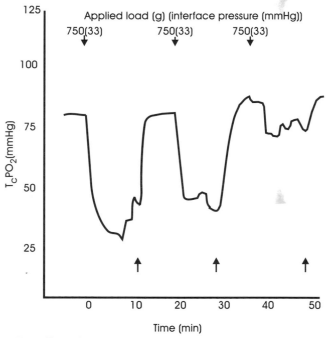

Figure 2.2: The effect of repetitive loading — normal reaction
TcPO2 = *Transcutaneous oxygen tension*
Reproduced from Bader (1990) by kind permission of the publishers

Few prevalence surveys have assessed patients with pressure sores for neurological problems. Dealey (1994) found it to be a significant factor for 48.6% of patients in a survey carried out in 1989 and for 35.7% of patients in a 1993 survey. Claus-Walker *et al* (1973) found a reduced level of collagen in the dermis of spinal cord injured patients. Bader (1990) found that some patients with spinal injury or neurological disease appeared to have an abnormal response to repetitive loading. The normal response is reactive hyperaemia and a vasomotor response which assists in maintaining tissue oxygen levels during subsequent loading (*Figure 2.2*). *Figure 2.3* shows the results for a man with multiple sclerosis where repetitive loading resulted in gradually diminishing oxygen levels. Kabagambe *et al* (1994) carried out a similar study comparing 10 patients with spinal cord injury with 11 healthy subjects. They also found

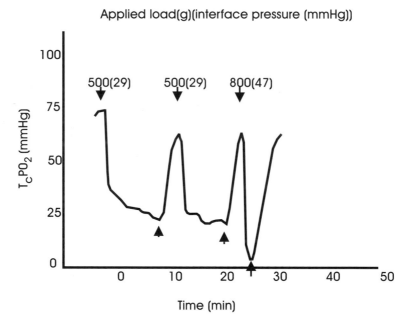

Figure 2-3: An abnormal response to repetitive loading
T_cPO_2 = *transcutaneous partial pressure of oxygen*
Reproduced from Bader (1990) by kind permission of the publishers

impaired reactive hyperaemia in the spinal cord injured patients. Obviously, an individual with this type of impaired response is at considerable risk of developing pressure sores.

Another intrinsic factor is poor oxygen perfusion in the tissues. This may occur as a result of heart disease, peripheral vascular disease, diabetes or the use of drugs that cause vasoconstriction. Whatever the cause, the local capillary closing pressure is lowered and has less resistance to pressure. The surrounding tissue is vulnerable as it lacks oxygen and essential nutrients.

A poor nutritional intake is considered to be associated with pressure sore development. Pinchcofsky-Devin and Kaminski (1986) assessed the nutritional status of 232 nursing home patients. They found that 117 had mild to moderate malnutrition and a further 17 were severely malnourished. The latter group all had pressure sores, whereas none of the other patients were affected. In a study of intrinsic factors related to pressure sore development in elderly people, Cullum and Clark (1992) found that patients with pressure sores had a significantly lower serum protein concentration than those without pressure sores. Berlowitz and Wilking (1989) studied 299 patients in a chronic care hospital. They compared the nutritional intake of 100 patients admitted with pressure sores with that of 199 admitted without pressure sores. They found that impaired nutritional intake was significantly associated with the presence of pressure sores and also with the development of new sores. Goode *et al* (1992) found an association between vitamin C depletion and pressure sore development in a group of elderly patients with fractured neck of femur.

Certainly malnutrition and also dehydration reduce the elasticity of the tissues. The collagen content of the dermis can also be affected. Prolonged malnutrition leads to anaemia and tissue hypoxia.

Body weight may also be a factor in pressure sore development. Very thin or emaciated patients have little padding over the bony prominences and are therefore much more vulnerable to pressure. Equally, obese patients may also be more vulnerable. Despite the use of a variety of aids, it may be difficult to move such patients without dragging them up the bed or chair.

Incontinence has also been demonstrated to be a factor in pressure sore development. Fletcher (1992) reviewed the epidemiology of pressure sores and found that incontinence was often associated with pressure sores. Kelly (1994) suggested that the risk of pressure sore development can be increased fivefold by the presence of even small amounts of moisture. Jordan and Clark (1977) surveyed 10 751 patients and found a pressure sore incidence of 20.7% among incontinent patients compared with only 3.7% among continent patients. Brandeis *et al* (1994) studied 4232 nursing home residents and found that faecal incontinence was a high risk factor in nursing homes with a high incidence of pressure sores.

Major surgery may be a factor in pressure damage. Dealey (1994) found that it was the most common factor in tissue breakdown, affecting 64.3% of patients. Hicks (1971) found a pressure sore incidence of 13% in surgical patients and Stotts (1988) an incidence of 17%. An in-depth study of surgical patients by Kemp (1990) found that elderly patients undergoing lengthy operations that involved the use of an extracorporeal circulation were the most vulnerable.

It has also been suggested that acute illness is a factor in pressure sore development. Anecdotal evidence has shown that the usual prevention strategies for the long-term at-risk patient are ineffective if the patient becomes ill. Bliss (1990) proposed that the acutely ill are especially vulnerable, possibly because of heart failure, vasomotor failure, vasoconstriction due to shock, pain, low blood pressure or other factors. Allman *et al* (1995) studied 286 patients admitted to a teaching hospital. All were confined to bed or a chair for at least 5 days. Thirty-seven patients (12.9%) developed pressure sores. Of these, 56.8% developed sores within the first 2 weeks of their admission, ie. at the time when they were most ill.

A pressure sore may also be an indication that the patient is terminally ill. Eckman (1989) suggested that 25% of corpses in funeral homes in the USA have pressure sores. Hanson *et al* (1991) studied hospice patients and found that 62% of pressure sores developed in the last 2 weeks of life. Bliss (1993) reported that patients with advanced disease may suddenly develop deep necrotic pressure sores in the 1 or 2 weeks before death. Such sores may develop despite the use of previously effective prevention strategies.

External factors

A number of external factors may exacerbate some of the extrinsic or intrinsic factors. Inappropriate positioning may increase the risk of tissue damage due to pressure or shear. For example, inappropriate positioning of a stroke patient may encourage the patient to fall to one side when sitting in a chair. This has the effect of considerably increasing the pressure over one ischial tuberosity. If the patient is then left in that position for some time, pressure damage is likely to occur.

Another factor to consider is external restraint to movement. The use of restraining garments is considered unacceptable in the UK, although such garments are widely used in North America. Obviously, the use of restraining garments prevents movement and precludes pressure relief. But it is not just restraining garments that can restrict the ability to move. A patient lying on a trolley may be frightened to move for fear of falling, or be unable to move because of the narrow surface. Unfortunately, patients may be left on trolleys for long periods, eg. while waiting to be warded. Versluysen (1986) reported trolley waits ranging from 54 minutes to 12 hours 30 minutes with a median of 3 hours 15 minutes. Patients may be expected to lie in one position for long periods when undergoing investigations, such as complex X-rays. During this time, they may have to lie on very hard surfaces.

Equally, poor lifting and handling techniques may increase the risk of shear or friction. Poor lifting may result in a patient sliding down in the bed or chair. It may also cause the patient to be dragged rather than lifted clear of the supporting surface.

Inappropriate clothing may also be a problem. This may be especially relevant to those with loss of sensation as well as poor mobility. Trousers with stiff seams such as jeans can cause problems for those confined to a wheelchair. The seams can cause localised pressure. The advent of the tracksuit as a fashion garment has been beneficial to wheelchair users. Tight shoes can also cause pressure problems. Classically, diabetics are vulnerable to this type of problem, but anyone with loss of sensation could also have difficulties with tight shoes, especially those with oedema.

Drugs have an important role in the management of many conditions. However, they can also increase a patient's risk of developing pressure sores. Sedatives and hypnotics may make the patient excessively sleepy and thus reduce mobility. Ineffective pain control can also reduce mobility as the patient may keep still in a bid to reduce the pain.

Finally, poor hygiene may result in a patient lying in a pool of urine or in faeces for excessively long periods. Equally, failure to wash the sweaty patient can also result in the patient sitting or lying in excessive moisture. As has already been noted, moisture increases friction forces.

Comment

The potential causes of pressure sores are summarised in *Table 2.1*. It can be seen that the causes of pressure sore development are extremely complex and, as yet, poorly understood.

Table 2.1: The causes of pressure sores.

Extrinsic factors	Pressure
	Friction
	Shear
Intrinsic factors	Age
	Reduced mobility
	Neurological deficit
	Poor oxygen perfusion
	Poor nutrition
	Emaciation/obesity
	Incontinence
	Acute illness
	Terminal illness
External factors	Inappropriate positioning
	External restraints to movement
	Poor lifting and handling techniques
	Inappropriate clothing
	Drugs
	Poor hygiene

Key points

1. Pressure sores are caused by a combination of intrinsic, extrinsic and external factors

2. Pressure is the most important factor in pressure sore development

3. The causes of pressure sores are not completely understood

References

Allman RM, Goode PS, Patrick MM, Burst N, Bartolucci AA (1995) Pressure ulcer risk factors among hospitalised patients with activity limitation. *JAMA* **273**(11): 865–70

Bader D (1990) Compressive Loading Effects on Tissue Viability. In: Bader D, ed. *Pressure Sores — Clinical Practice and Scientific Approach*. Macmillan Press, London: 191–201

Berlowitz DR, Wilking SVB (1989) Risk factors for pressure sores: a comparison of cross-sectional and cohort-derived data. *J Am Geriatr Soc* **37**(11): 1043–50

Bliss M (1990) Preventing pressure sores. (Editorial). *Lancet* **335**: 1311–12

Bliss M (1993) Aetiology of pressure sores. *Rev Clin Gerontol* **3**: 379–97

Brandeis GH, Ooi WL, Hossain M, Morris JN, Lipsitz LA (1994) A longitudinal study of risk factors associated with the formation of pressure ulcers in nursing homes. *J Am Geriatr Soc* **42**: 388–93

Bridel J (1993) The aetiology of pressure sores. *J Wound Care* **2**(4): 230–8

Claus-Walker J, Campos RJ, Carter RE, Chapman M (1973) Electrolytes in urinary calculi and urine of patients with spinal cord injuries. *Arch Phys Med Rehabil* **54**: 109–14

Cullum N, Clark M (1992) Intrinsic factors associated with pressure sores in elderly people. *J Adv Nurs* **17**: 427–31

David J, Chapman RG, Chapman EJ, Lockett B (1983) *An Investigation of the Current Methods used in Nursing for the Care of Patients with Established Pressure Sores*. Nursing Practice Research Unit, Northwick Park, London

Dealey C (1994) Monitoring the pressure sore problem in a teaching hospital. *J Adv Nurs* **20**: 652–9

Eckman KL (1989) The prevalence of dermal ulcers among persons who have died. *Decubitus* **2**(2): 36–40

Fletcher A (1992) The epidemiology of two common age-related wounds. *J Wound Care* **1**(4): 39–43

Gebhardt K (1995) What causes pressure sores? *Nurs Stand* **9**(Suppl 31): 48–51

Goode HF, Burns E, Walker BE (1992) Vitamin C depletion and pressure sores in elderly patients with femoral neck fracture. *Br Med J* **305**: 925–6

Hall DA, Reed FB, Nuki G *et al* (1974) The relative effects of age and corticosteroid therapy on the collagen profiles of dermis from subjects with rheumatoid arthritis. *Age Ageing* **3**: 15

Hall DA, Blackett AD, Zajac AR *et al* (1981) Changes in skin fold thickness with increasing age. *Age Ageing* **10**: 19

Hanson D, Langemo DK, Olson B *et al* (1991) The prevalence and incidence of pressure ulcers in the hospice setting: analysis of two methodologies. *Am J Hospice Palliat Care* **5**: 18–22

Hicks DJ (1971) *An Incidence Study of Pressure Sores Following Surgery.* ANA Clinical Sessions: 1970 Miami. Appleton-Century-Crofts, New York: 49–54

Jordan MM, Clark M (1977) *Report on the Incidence of PRrssure Sores in the Patient Community of the Greater Glasgow Health Board Area.* University of Strathclyde, Glasgow

Kabagambe MK, Swain I, Shakespeare P (1994) An investigation of the effects on the microcirculation of the skin (reactive hyperaemia) in spinal cord injured patients. *J Tissue Viabil* **4**(4): 110–23

Kelly J (1994 The aetiology of pressure sores. *J Tissue Viabil* **4**(3): 77–8

Kemp M (1990) Factors that contribute to pressure sores in surgical patients. *Res Nurs Health* **13**: 293–301

Krouskop TA (1978) Mechanisms of decubitus ulcer formation — an hypothesis. *Med Hypotheses* **4**(1): 37–9

Landis EM (1931) Micro-injection studied of capillary blood pressure in human skin. *Heart* **15**: 209–28

Pinchcofski-Devin G, Devin MV (1986) Correlation of pressure sores and nutritional status. *J Am Geriatr Soc* **34**: 435–40

Schubert V (1992) Hypotension as risk factor for the development of pressure sores in elderly patients. *J Tissue Viabil* **2**(1): 5–8

Stotts NA (1988) Predicting pressure ulcer development in surgical patients. *Heart Lung* **17**: 641–7

Versluysen M (1986) How elderly patients with femoral fractures develop pressure sores in hospital. *Br Med J* **292**: 1311–13

Chapter 3
Risk assessment

Introduction

A major aspect of pressure sore prevention is the correct identification of those at risk of pressure sore development. Wilson (1995) defines risk as 'the potential for an unwanted or unexpected outcome'. She describes a number of clinical risks, one of which is 'patient injury while in the provider's care resulting in extensive resource utilisation to correct injury'. Pressure sores certainly fit into that category.

Risk assessment can be seen as a form of clinical risk modification which will lower the potential for healthcare risk. A draft of national Clinical Practice Guidelines for the Prevention and Management of Pressure Sores (Collinson and Hitch, 1995) suggest that the assessment of risk should be part of a comprehensive patient assessment. In other words, all patients in vulnerable areas should be assessed routinely. This may not be appropriate in areas such as acute psychiatry, obstetrics and paediatrics.

Once a patient is identified as being at risk, appropriate preventive measures should be implemented. Failure to do so could be seen as negligence. All healthcare professionals have a duty of care to their patients. Negligence is a failure in the duty of care owed to another, eg. a patient, with resultant harm to that person (Young, 1995). Merely recording the degree of risk of a patient and taking no further action is a failure to take due care.

The frequency of risk assessment

Risk assessment should be seen as a dynamic process. Most patients' conditions do not remain static. Patients should be reassessed when their condition alters. The frequency of routine assessment will vary according to the clinical area. Within surgical wards it may be appropriate to assess patients once before surgery and then daily until they are no longer at risk. In other acute areas, patients may need to be assessed daily from admission. In chronic areas, such as elderly care or rehabilitation units, where changes in patient condition are usually much slower, a weekly assessment is more likely to be appropriate. In the community, a monthly assessment is probably adequate or even 3-monthly in some cases.

There are no hard-and-fast rules for the frequency of risk assessment. Certainly there is no research evidence to provide guidance. A pragmatic approach would be to establish the practice of routine assessment, the frequency of which would depend on the patient group, with the recognition of the need to undertake more frequent assessment in the event of changes in an individual patient's condition.

The elements of risk assessment

The draft of the national Clinical Practice Guidelines (Collinson and Hitch, 1995) suggests that a number of factors are involved in the assessment of pressure sore risk. They are:

- Assessment of skin
- Assessment of the general condition of the patient
- Relevant history of mental and physical health
- A calculation of risk

Assessment of skin

Regular assessment of the skin, especially over bony prominences, is essential for the early identification of pressure problems. Persistent redness over an area indicates the need to take immediate remedial action. Note should also be taken of fragile skin and areas of scar tissue from previous pressure damage. Healthcare assistants have an important role in skin assessment. They should be trained to automatically assess the bony prominences of patients when attending to their hygiene needs and to report any problems to a trained nurse.

Assessment of the general condition of the patient

The draft of the national Clinical Practice Guidelines suggests that assessment of the general condition of the patient should include their medical condition (Collinson and Hitch, 1995). This is because particular diagnoses have been found to predispose the sufferer to pressure sore development. One example is fractured neck of femur. Versluysen (1986) found a pressure sore incidence of 66% in this patient group.

Relevant history of mental and physical health

The intrinsic factors that can predispose an individual to pressure sore development are discussed in chapter 2. A patient history will aid identification of any relevant intrinsic factors. This might include previous pressure damage, loss of sensation or neuropathy in parts of the body, reduced mobility, poor motivation etc. Identification of any specific problems will assist in the development of an appropriate plan of care.

Calculation of risk

There are a number of scoring systems which allow the nurse to calculate the degree of risk of an individual patient. The earliest was that published by Norton first in 1962 and later in 1975 (Norton *et al*, 1962; 1975). When Norton began her seminal work into the problems of elderly patients in hospital, she developed a research tool to assist in identifying patients at risk of developing pressure sores. This became known as the Norton Score and was a new concept in providing a mathematical method for calculating pressure sore risk (*Figure 3.1*).

SCORING SYSTEM KEY: TOTAL SCORE OF 14 or below = 'AT RISK'				
A Physical condition	**B** Mental condition	**C** Activity	**D** Mobility	**E** Incontinent
Good 4	Alert 4	Ambulant 4	Full 4	Not 4
Fair 3	Apathetic 3	Walk/help 3	Slightly limited 3	Occasion-ally 3
Poor 2	Confused 2	Chair-bound 2	Very limited 2	Usually urine 2
Very bad 1	Stuporous 1	Bedfast 1	Immobile 1	Doubly 1

Figure 3.1: The Norton Score

The concept of a risk calculator involves taking a number of factors relevant to pressure damage and breaking them down into degrees of severity. Each degree of severity is given a score. The patient is assessed and given a score for each factor. The scores are then added together to obtain the degree of risk of the patient. For example, the factors used in the Norton Score are physical condition, mental condition, activity, mobility and incontinence.

During the 1980s, the concept of using a risk calculator in patient assessment became widely acknowledged. A number of criticisms were made of the Norton Score, which led to the development of other risk calculators. The most frequent criticism of the Norton Score is that it was developed for use with elderly patients and is not necessarily suitable for younger groups (Chapman and Chapman, 1986). Lincoln *et al* (1986) found limitations in the validity and reliability of the Norton Score. Validity relates to the predictive ability of a scoring system to correctly identify those who will develop sores. Interrater reliability relates to the frequency with which different nurses agree on the score for a specific patient.

Some of the more widely known scoring systems will be described, indicating the patient group for whom each one was developed, the variables used in the score and the scoring system.

Norton Score (Norton et al, 1975)

Care group: Elderly patients

Variables used: Physical health, mental health, activity, mobility and incontinence

Scoring system: The lower the score the higher the risk. Maximum score 20; score of 14 or below indicates patient at risk

Knoll Score (Abruzzese, 1982)

Care group: Acute care patients

Variables used: General state of health, mental status, activity, mobility, incontinence, oral nutritional intake, oral fluid intake, predisposing diseases (diabetes, neuropathies, vascular disease, anaemia)

Scoring system: The higher the score the higher the risk. Highest score 33; scores above 12 indicate patient at risk

Waterlow Score *(Waterlow, 1985)*

Care group: Acute care patients

Variables used: Build/weight for height, continence, skin type, mobility, sex, age, appetite, tissue malnutrition, neurological deficit, major surgery/trauma, medication

Scoring system: The higher the score the higher the risk. Scores divided into categories:

10–14 = at risk;
15–19 = high risk;
20+ = very high risk

Douglas Score *(Pritchard, 1986)*

Care group: General medical ward patients

Variables: Nutritional state/haemoglobin, activity, incontinence, pain, skin state, mental state, special risk factors (diabetes, steroid therapy, cytotoxic therapy, dyspnoea)

Scoring system: The lower the score the higher the risk. Highest score 24; scores below 18 indicate patient at risk

Braden Score *(Bergstrom et al, 1987)*

Care group: Nursing home patients

Variables: Sensory perception, moisture, activity, mobility, nutrition, friction and shear

Scoring system: The lower the score the higher the risk. Highest score 23, indicating low risk; lowest score 6, indicating high risk

Lowthian Score or Pressure Sore Prediction Scale Score
(Lowthian, 1987)

Care group: Orthopaedic patients

Variables: Sitting up, unconscious, poor general condition, incontinence, mobility

Scoring system: The higher the score the higher the risk. Highest score 16; scores above 6 indicate patient at risk

Walsall Community Pressure Sore Risk Calculator (Milward, 1993)

Care group: Community patients

Variables: Predisposing disease, level of consciousness, mobility, skin condition, nutritional status, pain, bladder incontinence, bowel incontinence, carer

Scoring system: The higher the score the higher the risk. The score is divided into risk categories:

3–5 = very low risk
6–11 = low risk
12–22 = medium risk
23–36 = high risk

There has recently been much discussion in the literature concerning the value of risk calculators. Some of the debate concerns the threshold score. This is the score at which the individual falls into the at-risk category. For example, for the Norton Score the threshold score is 14. Clark and Farrar (1992) studied six risk calculators and suggested that the threshold score between no risk and at risk was different from that cited in the literature. They proposed that a threshold score should be identified for each hospital or patient group. However, few people have the necessary skills to determine this. Bridel (1993) reviewed the literature to determine the validity and reliability of the Norton, Waterlow and Braden Scores. Bridel concluded that there were problems with each of these risk assessment tools: the Norton Score was unable to predict accurately; the Waterlow Score overpredicted; and, although the Braden Score has been more rigorously researched, the assessment has to be carried out by a registered nurse. The main difficulty in validating the usefulness of any risk calculator is that preventive measures would have to be suspended for the period of the research. This is totally unethical and cannot be done.

Conclusions

The main points regarding risk assessment and the use of risk calculators are listed in the Key Points. Good patient assessment will ensure that patients at risk of developing pressure sores are correctly identified. This will result in effective use of limited resources.

Key points

1.   The risk calculator selected for use should be appropriate for the patient group

2.   A risk calculator should assist clinical judgment, not be a substitute for it

3.   A single assessment on admission is not adequate; it should be ongoing, reflecting changes in the patient's condition

4.   Assessment of risk should include assessment of skin, general condition, relevant past history and calculation of risk

5.   Identification of risk should result in the development of an appropriate prevention plan

6.   Failure to take due care constitutes negligence

References

Abruzzese RS (1982) The effectiveness of an assessment tool in specifying nursing care to prevent decubitus ulcers. In: *PRN: The Adelphi Report: Project for Research in Nursing*. Adelphi University, Garden City, New York: 43–60

Bergstrom N, Braden B, Laguzza A (1987) The Braden scale for predicting pressure risk. *Nurs Res* **36**(4): 205–10

Bridel J (1993) Assessing the risk of pressure sores. *Nurs Stand* **7**(25): 32–5

Chapman EJ, Chapman R (1986) Treatment of pressure sores: the state of the art. In: Tierney AJ, ed. *Clinical Nursing Practice*. Churchill Livingstone, Edinburgh

Clark M, Farrar S (1992) Comparison of risk calculators. In: Harding KG, Leaper DL, Turner TD, eds. *Proceedings of the 1st European Conference on Advances in Wound Management*. Macmillan Magazines, London

Collinson G, Hitch S (1995) *Prevention and Management of Pressure Sores: Clinical Practice Guidelines*. Draft Guideline Synopsis. Clinical Effectiveness from Guidelines to Cost-effective Practice Conference, 3–4 May. London

Lincoln R, Roberts R, Maddox A, Levine S, Patterson C (1986) Use of the Norton pressure sore risk assessment scoring system with elderly patients in acute care. *J Enterostomal Ther* **13**: 132–8

Lowthian P (1987) The practical assessment of pressure sore risk. *Care Sci Pract* **5**(4): 3–7

Milward P (1993) Scoring pressure sore risk in the community. *Nurs Stand* **3**(8): 50–5

Norton D, McLaren R, Exton-Smith AN (1962) *An Investigation of Geriatric Nursing Problems in Hospital*. National Corporation for the Care of Old People, London

Norton D, Exton-Smith AN, McLaren R (1975) *An Investigation of Geriatric Nursing Problems in Hospital*. Churchill

Livingstone, Edinburgh

Pritchard V (1986) Calculating the risk. *Nurs Times* **82**(8): 59–61

Versluysen M (1986) How elderly patients with femoral fracture develop pressure sores in hospital. *Br Med J* **292**: 1311–13

Waterlow J (1985) A risk assessment card. *Nurs Times* **81**(48): 49–55

Wilson J (1995) Clinical risk modification. *Br J Nurs* **4**(11): 667

Young A (1995) Negligence. *Br J Nurs* **4**(2): 119

Chapter 4

Pressure sore prevention strategies

Introduction

Once a patient has been assessed to be at risk of pressure sore development, an appropriate prevention plan should be drawn up. An understanding of the causes of pressure sores and the specific risk factors for the individual patient should inform the planning process. Successful prevention strategies require a multidisciplinary approach. This chapter discusses a range of preventive measures which will require input from varying members of the multidisciplinary team. Not all of these measures are necessary for every patient.

Prevention strategies

Pressure relief

If pressure is the major cause of pressure sores, then it follows that the relief of pressure is a major strategy in any prevention plan. This can be achieved by regular repositioning of a patient.

Traditionally, patients have been turned from side to side every 2 hours, often described as '2-hourly turning'. There is an apocryphal story that 2-hourly turning originated at East

Grinstead Hospital during the Second World War. When some of the severely injured airmen started to develop pressure sores, the surgeon in charge decided that they should be turned from side to side as a preventive measure. Three teams of orderlies working in shifts were given the task of going round the hospital turning the patients. It took 2 hours to complete one circuit of patients.

Currently, it is not always possible to achieve 2-hourly turning of patients. In the community it is impractical to even consider the possibility, except in exceptional circumstances. While it is more feasible in the hospital setting, the reduction in staffing levels in many areas makes it difficult to maintain strict 2-hourly turning throughout the 24-hour period.

Although the concept of 2-hourly turning persists and is often included in care plans, it is not necessary or suitable for all patients. Bliss (1990) suggests that many older people are not able to lie on their sides, perhaps because of cardiac or respiratory disease. Those with arthritis may find certain positions painful. Also, although patients sitting in chairs may still be at risk, they can hardly be turned from side to side.

It would seem that the term 'repositioning' is much more suitable. At present there is no evidence to indicate how frequently patients should be repositioned. Frequency of repositioning should be based on individual need and consideration of the surface upon which the patient is sitting or lying. Kosiak (1959) found that pressure damage could result from a surface exerting a high pressure over a short period of time or a lower pressure over a longer period of time. Thus, a patient sitting on a wheelchair canvas with an interface pressure in excess of 150 mmHg could only do so safely for a short period of time. If a cushion was placed in the chair, considerably reducing the interface pressure, the safe period would be extended.

Patients with spinal cord injuries are often taught to make frequent small movements to relieve pressure. Exton Smith and Sherwin (1961) measured the frequency with which elderly patients moved in their sleep. They found a strong relationship between the incidence of pressure sores and the inverse number of movements, ie. the fewer the movements, the higher the incidence of pressure sores. Most of these movements were fairly small, which suggests that small alterations in pressure can be effective. Thus, where patients are able, they can be taught to provide a certain amount of pressure relief for themselves.

Skin assessment

Although assessment of the skin, especially the bony prominences, is an essential part of the assessment process, it is also a preventive measure. Regular assessment of those parts of the body most at risk will enable any early indication of pressure damage to be detected. This can assist in determining the frequency with which repositioning should be carried out and the effectiveness of any pressure-relieving equipment that is being used.

Use of the 30° tilt position

As discussed previously, it is not possible to turn some patients from side to side. It is also not always possible to move some patients for long periods of time. Examples include the critically ill patient who is too unstable to move or the immobile patient living at home. The community services are rarely able to supply any input during the night and it is unreasonable to expect carers to do so. They may be elderly or in employment and are not able to cope with constantly broken nights. It follows that other means must be found to prevent pressure sore development.

A very useful method is the 30° tilt. It is simple to use and also very cheap, requiring only three pillows. Preston (1988) described the development of this method in a unit for younger disabled patients. It reduced the frequency of repositioning to 4-hourly for most patients and allowed some to have 8 hours uninterrupted sleep at night. This has clear benefits for the long-term at-risk patient.

Figure 4.1 shows how to place a patient into the 30° tilt position. The pelvis is tilted through 30°. When the patient is in this position, there is no pressure on the sacrum or heels. The greatest pressure is over the gluteal region of the buttocks. Preston (1988) found that this pressure was around 26 mmHg which is low enough to allow the patient to lie in this position for some time.

Another advantage of the 30° tilt position is that the patient can be moved from one buttock to the other without being lifted. The pillow can simply be slipped out and the patient rolled slightly to allow it to be inserted under the other side. This is very useful for critically ill patients as pressure relief can be provided with very little movement.

When the 30° tilt is instigated for long-term at-risk patients, the frequency of repositioning should be monitored carefully. As the time between moves is gradually extended, the pressure areas should be observed for signs of persistent hyperaemia. Ideally, this should be carried out in a hospital environment as part of the discharge planning. Ultimately, the nurses should be able to leave the patient at night for the length of time that he/she will be left after discharge. This will either confirm that the plan is effective, or indicate the need for a change of strategy.

The 30° tilt is not suitable for all patients. If the patient has contractures, he/she may not be able to straighten the legs adequately. Some patients who have muscle spasm cannot tolerate it. Although it can be used for those who need to sit upright, many of these patients cannot tolerate the tilt. However, it is a useful adjunct to care and is very helpful for suitable patients.

Reductions of shear and friction

A wide-ranging view is needed when considering how to

Use of the 30° tilt position

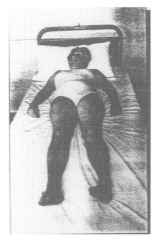

The 30° Tilt is a useful method for positioning patients who are difficult to turn or are not able to lie on their side. Patients may be safely left for long periods in this position, but the pressure areas should be carefully monitored to establish an appropriate time for each patient.

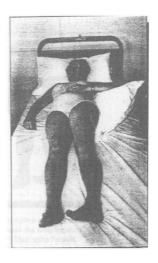

1 Place the patient in the centre of the bed with sufficient pillows to support the head and neck.

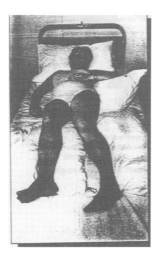

2 Place a pillow at an angle under one buttock thus tilting the pelvis by 30°. Check with a flattened hand that the sacrum is just clear of the mattress.

The patient may be turned by removing the pillow under the buttock and placing it under the other buttock.

This can be done by two nurses rolling the patient slightly. No lifting is necessary.

3 Place a pillow lengthways under each leg so that the heels are lifted clear of the bed.

Figure 4.1: 30° tilt position

reduce shear and friction in patients with restricted mobility. Patients with full mobility are less likely to have problems with shear and friction. Shear or friction can occur when the patient is in bed or sitting in a chair, or when the patient is being moved. This means that a number of factors have to be considered, such as the position of the patient in bed or on a chair and the methods being used to move the patient.

One problem is that the patient may slide down the bed or in the chair. This may be further exacerbated by the patient pulling him/herself up the bed, causing friction to heels and elbows. There are two strategies that may be tried to alleviate this problem. One is to try to prevent the patient sliding. Profiling beds can help or, if one is not available, slightly tilting the end of the bed may be effective. A foot board may be useful for some patients, but is not suitable for stroke patients as it can increase spasticity. It may also be necessary to review the type of seating being provided. The physiotherapist or occupational therapist will be able to provide advice regarding equipment. The other strategy is to protect the heels and elbows. Application of a film dressing can be a very effective way of preventing friction (Hall, 1983). The use of a monkey pole (when suitable) can be helpful as the patient can lift him/herself clear of the bed.

Friction and shear can also occur when the patient is moving in bed or from bed to chair. In the past, this may have occurred when a heavy patient was lifted ineffectively. The introduction of regulations concerning manual handling should now prevent this from happening (Health and Safety Executive, 1992). The availability of a variety of aids including hoists should reduce the risk of friction damage. However, it is important to ensure that the slings being used with a hoist are suitable for the patient, otherwise they may cut into the skin, especially on the thighs. If there is any uncertainty, advice can be sought from the manual handling trainer who can carry out a risk assessment and advise on suitable methods of handling a patient. Nurses should remember that they have a duty of care to themselves and their patients to use all reasonable care for their own safety and that of others (Royal College of Nursing, 1993). Transfer boards are a very effective means of enabling disabled patients to transfer from bed to chair or vice versa. However, they can be a source of shearing if used inappropriately. The board should have a smooth surface with no sharp edges. The patient should be able to lift him/herself across it bit by bit. If the patient is only able to slide, then it is best to use a sliding sheet with the board. Bath boards may be a source of tissue damage if they are slatted or poorly made with rough surfaces. The patient is expected to slide and twist across the surface. This could increase the likelihood of tissue damage in an at-risk patient. Again, advice can be sought from the therapist.

Nutritional support

Monitoring the nutritional status of patients should be part of the assessment process for all patients in hospital and vulnerable patients in the community. McWirter and Pennington (1994) assessed 500 patients on admission and found that 200 (40%) were undernourished.

Malnutrition occurs when an individual's dietary intake fails to meet his/her metabolic requirements. Factors that may be associated with reduced nutritional status are:

Acute illness: Often results in loss of appetite, although nutritional requirements may be increased

Chronic illness: Disease or the drug therapy may affect appetite or result in malabsorption

Pain: May result in loss of appetite

Age: Increases the risk of disease

Polypharmacy: May result in drug-related malnutrition

Physical disability: May cause difficulties in shopping, cooking or feeding

Mental disorder: Patient is less likely to be aware of the need for a good diet

Masticatory inefficiency: Patient may be unable to eat full range of foodstuffs

Alcoholism: Often associated with poor diet and can cause thiamine deficiency

Poverty: Often results in poor intake of protein and vitamins

Lack of care: In hospital, food may be placed out of reach, the patient may be left lying supine, or investigations or ward rounds may be carried out at meal times

As well as ascertaining whether a patient has a poor nutritional status, it is beneficial to try to identify the causative factors. For example, if a patient is hardly eating because he/she has arthritic hands and is unable to hold cutlery, it should be relatively easy to resolve the problem, whereas if a demented patient refuses to eat, it may be more problematic.

The dietitian will be able to assist in both assessing the individual needs of a patient and developing an appropriate management plan. Some patients may benefit from dietary supplements. Delmi *et al* (1990) showed that providing supplements for elderly patients with fractured neck of femur significantly reduced the incidence of complications and duration of hospital stay. This is important when the vulnerability of these patients to pressure sore development is considered. Penfold and Crowther (1989) suggested some practical ways to improve the dietary intake of the elderly. For example, the occupational therapist can provide guidance on suitably adapted cutlery for those with arthritic hands.

Patients who are unable to tolerate an oral diet may be tube fed. A suitable regimen can be planned by the dietitian. Only when enteral feeding is not possible should total parenteral nutrition (TPN) be considered. While it is certainly life-saving for some, TPN can also be hazardous with a risk of infection and, potentially, septicaemia (King's Fund Centre, 1992).

Skin care

Care of the skin of incontinent patients can be problematic. Constant washing can result in drying and a loss of skin resilience. Patients with severe diarrhoea may develop excoriation of the skin which can be very painful. Guidelines on pressure sore prevention produced by an American government agency, the Agency for Healthcare Policy and Research (1992), suggested that the use of a mild cleansing agent would help to reduce the risk of skin dryness and that a barrier cream would protect against loss of moisture. Byers *et al* (1994) found that the use of a cleanser and barrier cream resulted in a significantly lower loss of skin moisture than did the use of soap and water.

Although American nurses seem to have recognised the benefits of using a cleanser and barrier cream for incontinent patients, this may be less true of their British counterparts. Dealey (1995) found resistance to changing from using soap and water to the use of a cleanser and barrier cream. In her study, 38% of nurses questioned commented that soap and water was as effective if not better than a cleanser and barrier cream. Dealey postulated that the nursing staff involved in the study may have received inadequate training in this area, resulting in resistance to change.

Effective management of incontinence is an essential part of skin care as well as being important for patient dignity. A huge range of products are available, ranging from pads of all types to sophisticated urinary appliances and urethral catheters. The continence advisor can provide assistance in managing difficult continence problems.

Protecting the patient with neurological deficit

Patients who have loss of sensation are particularly vulnerable to localised pressure. This can be caused by inappropriate clothing with heavy seams or by tight shoes. Preventive strategies should include careful monitoring of the skin and advice on suitable clothing. As this is generally a chronic problem, patients should be taught to take as much responsibility for themselves as possible.

Patient education

It is important that patients are involved as much as possible in their plan of care. The degree of involvement will vary from patient to patient. Healthcare professionals should recognise that most patients, other than the totally immobile or unconscious, can take some responsibility for themselves. Patient education should be an essential part of the care plan. Whether patients are at short-term or long-term risk of developing pressure sores, they should be told why they are at risk and have the proposed preventive strategies explained to them. Written information can enhance oral explanation. A number of hospitals have produced their own explanatory booklets. The Department of Health has also produced a booklet for patients and carers, copies of which can be obtained free of charge (see page 115).

Patients at long-term risk need further education on how to assess their skin and an understanding of the preventive strategies and any equipment that might be used. They also need to understand the importance of taking extra precautions if they are unwell for any reason. As more patients with physical disability are cared for in the community, they will increasingly need a good understanding of their own healthcare needs. Equally, if they are subsequently admitted to hospital, nursing staff should take note of the patient's previous knowledge and experience.

Staff education

The draft of the national Clinical Practice Guidelines on Pressure Sore Prevention suggest that education is essential for the successful implementation of any policy or practice guidelines (Collinson and Hitch, 1995). It is also recognised that any educational programme should be multidisciplinary and an ongoing process. Moody *et al* (1988) demonstrated that the implementation of an educational programme in a hospital for the elderly assisted in reducing the incidence of pressure sores.

It must not be assumed that all healthcare professionals have adequate knowledge regarding the causes, prevention and management of pressure sores. Gould (1992) carried out a postal survey in 1985 in which questionnaires regarding the teaching relating to pressure sores at basic and post-basic levels were sent to 13 colleges of nursing. She was disappointed to find that the topic was given low priority. Prevention was discussed in introductory courses but not later in the course. The treatment of pressure sores was largely ignored, with a tendency to deny their existence. There seemed to be little interest in the inclusion of pressure sore prevention and management in continuing education courses or study days. Equally, Sutton and Wallace (1990) and Bennet (1992) found that doctors and medical students have a limited understanding of the topic, and tended to see pressure sores as a nursing problem.

Happily, there has been a much greater interest in pressure sores in the decade since Gould's survey. While this may not yet be reflected in basic training for nurses and doctors, it has been introduced to a greater extent into post-registration education. There are a number of tissue viability courses available around the country and numerous study days and conferences.

Discharge planning

There has been a greater emphasis on planning for the discharge of patients from hospital since the introduction of care in the community. Before any patient who is at long-term risk of developing pressure sores is discharged, an effective package of care should be established for the individual patient. It is no use assuming that relatives can turn a patient at intervals through the night each night for evermore. Such a situation will only result in exhaustion for the carer, possible damage to relationships and a failed discharge.

Ideally, a suitable surface or position (such as the 30° tilt) on which the patient can safely lie all night should be established. The night staff are essential in assisting in this part of discharge planning. Their role is to gradually reduce the frequency of repositioning the patient while constantly monitoring the pressure areas for any indications of prolonged redness. If there are problems, an alternative solution will have to be considered. If all is well, the patient and carer will be able to feel confident that they can manage successfully after discharge.

If the patient is likely to be sitting in a chair for long periods, appropriate seating will be needed. A home visit involving the patient, carer, occupational therapist and other members of the healthcare team will assist in identifying further equipment needs.

Other aspects of care must also be considered, including appropriate education for both patient and carer. Where poor nutrition has been a factor in pressure sore development, strategies may be needed to ensure an adequate diet after discharge. Advice can be obtained from the dietitian. The community liaison sister can provide assistance in planning an appropriate package of care as well as communicating with the district nursing team. Clear information should be provided regarding the position, grade and treatment of any pressure sores.

Conclusion

There is a wide range of strategies that can be used to prevent pressure sore development. So far, the use of pressure-relieving equipment has not been discussed. This is such a large topic that it requires a chapter of its own.

Key points

1. Regular repositioning is an important preventive measure

2. The frequency of repositioning is dependent on several factors:
    - the patient's physical ability to cope with different positions
    - the surface on which the patient is sitting or lying
    - regular assessment of the bony prominences

3. The 30° tilt is a useful adjunct to care

4. The risk of tissue damage due to friction and shear can be reduced by providing effective means of assisting movement in bed and chair or between the two

5. Patients should be assessed for their nutritional status and support given when required

6. The use of a cleanser and barrier cream can help to reduce dryness and loss of skin resilience in the incontinent patient

7. The education of both patients and staff should be an essential part of any prevention strategy

8. All patients at long-term risk of developing pressure sores should have an appropriate package of care planned before discharge from hospital

References

Agency for healthcare Policy and Research (1992) *Pressure Ulcers in Adults: Prediction and Prevention.* AHCPR, Rockville

Bennet G (1992) Medical undergraduate teaching in chronic wound care (a survey). *J Tissue Viabil* **2(2)**: 50–1

Bliss M (1990) Geriatric Medicine. In: Bader D, ed. *Pressure Sores — Clinical Practice and Scientific Approach.* Macmillan Press, London: 65–80

Byers PH, Ryan PA, Shields A (1994) Effect of incontinence care cleansing regimes on skin integrity. Paper presented at Wound Ostomy and Continence Society Meeting, Baltimore, June

Collinson G, Hitch S (1995) Prevention and Management of Pressure Sores, Clinical Practice Guidelines. Guideline Synopsis. Clinical Effectiveness: From Guidelines to Cost-Effective Practice Conference, May 3–4. London

Dealey C (1995) Pressure sores and incontinence: a study evaluating the use of topical agents in skin care. *J Wound Care* **4(3)**: 103–5

Delmi M, Rapin C-H, Bengoa J-M, Delmas PD, Vasey H, Bonjour J-P (1990) Dietary supplementation in elderly patients with fractured neck of femur. *Lancet* **335**: 1013–16

Exton Smith AN, Sherwin RW (1961) The prevention of pressure sores: significance of spontaneous bodily movements. *Lancet* **ii**: 1124–5

Gould D (1992) Teaching students about pressure sores. *Nurs Stand* **6(26)**: 28–31

Hall P (1983) Prophylactic use of Opsite on pressure areas. *Nurs Focus* Jan/Feb

Health and Safety Executive (1992) *Manual Handling Operations Regulations.* HMSO, London

King's Fund Centre (1992) *A Positive Approach to Nutrition as Treatment.* King's Fund Centre, London

Kosiak M (1959) Etiology and pathology of ischemic ulcers. *Arch Phys Med Rehabil* **40**: 62–9

McWirter JP, Pennington C (1994) Incidence and recognition of malnutrition in hospital. *Br Med J* **308**: 945–8

Moody B, Fanale J, Thompson M, Vaillancourt D, Symonds G, Bonasoro C (1988) Impact of staff education on pressure sore development in elderly hospitalised patients. *Arch Intern Med* **148**(10): 2241–3

Penfold P, Crowther S (1989) Causes and management of neglected diet in the elderly. *Care Elderly* **1**(1): 20–2

Preston K (1988) Positioning for comfort and pressure relief: the 30 degree alternative. *Care Sci Pract* **6**(4): 116–19

Royal College of Nursing (1993) *Code of Practice for the Handling of Patients*. RCN, London

Sutton J, Wallace W (1990) Pressure sores: the views and practices of senior hospital doctors. *Care Sci Pract* **8**(3): 115–18

Chapter 5
The use of pressure-relieving equipment

Introduction

The range of strategies that may be used to prevent pressure sores were discussed in Chapter 4. This chapter moves the discussion on to the range of equipment that may be used as part of the prevention plan. The various types of equipment are listed in *Table 5.1*.

Table 5.1: The different types of pressure-relieving equipment

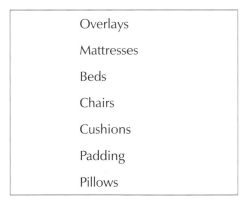

Overlays
Mattresses
Beds
Chairs
Cushions
Padding
Pillows

The use of pressure-relieving equipment is a useful adjunct to the main preventive measure of regular repositioning. A report by the Royal College of Physicians (1986) called for an adequate supply of pressure-relieving equipment to be available for those patients at risk of pressure sores. Hibbs (1990) put forward suggestions as to the range and amount of equipment that might be needed in a large health district for both hospital and community patients during one year.

There are large numbers of pressure-relieving and pressure-reducing mattresses and beds available for purchase or for rental. For those who have to make decisions about appropriate purchase, the situation can be very confusing. Each manufacturer provides information about the appropriate usage of their own equipment. However, there is a dearth of information about the effectiveness of the equipment. Young (1992a) surveyed the manufacturers of 48 different products asking for evidence of effectiveness. He found the results disappointing. Twenty-four (50%) had no validating information and in 10 cases (21%) the evidence was purely anecdotal. A further 10 (21%) had undergone laboratory interface pressure evaluation. Only four (8%) had undergone any form of clinical trial and of these only two had been a randomised controlled trial. A review by Hitch (1995) found only 13 randomised controlled trials of pressure-relieving equipment. A recent *Effective Health Care Bulletin, The Prevention and Treatment of Pressure Sores* (University of Leeds, 1995) stated that 'there is insufficient research evidence on clinical or cost-effectiveness to guide equipment choice.'

So is there any justification for using such expensive equipment? Bliss and Thomas (1992) admitted that, at the time of writing, their health authority budget for pressure relieving equipment was overspent by £70 000, and that the total budget for hiring equipment had been spent on 0.6% of the patients. Clark and Cullum (1992) found that the prevalence of pressure sores in one health district had increased from 6.8% to 14.2% over a 4-year period, despite an increase in the availability of pressure-redistributing mattresses. They suggested that there could be a number of reasons for this: there was still insufficient equipment to

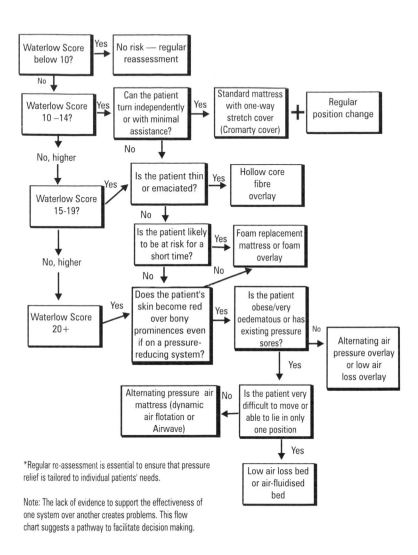

Figure 5-1: Flow chart for selecting mattresses*

Assessing support systems

Young (1992b) proposed a number of criteria by which support systems can be assessed or selected for use. This can be very helpful when there is a huge range of equipment from which to choose. An informal survey of current equipment identified over 70 different brand names, which can be divided into 18 different categories, for example foam overlay.

Young's criteria are as follows:

Effectiveness: This is the single most important criteria. If equipment is not effective it is no use. So the first question to ask is: does the equipment prevent pressure sores and is it suitable for the individual patient?

Ease of use: If equipment is easy to use, it is more likely to be acceptable to the nursing staff. It is also more likely to be used correctly.

Maintenance: Most support systems are in constant or frequent use. They need to be reliable and easy to maintain and repair.

Ease of nursing procedures: It is important that the system allows nurses to carry out procedures, such as washing or moving the patient, easily and safely.

Patient acceptability: The patient should find the system comfortable and not too hot or cold or too noisy. It should be remembered that the patient may not have any respite from the system.

Cost: Nurses have a responsibility to consider cost. It is not the most important factor when choosing a support system, but must be taken into consideration.

These criteria form the framework for *Table 5.2* which summarises information about the different types of overlays, mattresses and beds.

Effectiveness	Ease of use	Maintenance	Ease of nursing procedures	Patient acceptability	Cost (£)
Hollow core fibre overlays					
Suitable for low risk patients	Good	Laundering can result in matting of fibres	Not so easy moving patient in bed	Generally good	80–150
Foam overlays					
Good pressure reduction — for low to medium risk patients	Good	No problems	Generally good — raises height of bed — consideration with transfers	Generally good	50–100
Gel overlays					
Only demonstrated for operating table use	Heavy to move	None required	No problems	May find it cold to touch	150–300
Static air overlays					
Suitable for medium to high risk patients	Must be correct-ly inflated	Vulnerable to punctures	Generally no problems	Generally good	50–500
Alternating pressure air overlays					
Suitable for medium to high risk patients	Some training needed, but fairly simple to use	Annual maintenance check	Generally no problems — raises height of bed	Mostly good — some find movement unpleasant	700–2000
Low air loss overlays					
Suitable for medium to high risk patients	Some training needed, but fairly simple to use	Equipment most often rented	Generally no problems	Some find the pump noisy	–

Table 5.2: Assessing overlays, mattresses and beds

Effectiveness	Ease of use	Maintenance	Ease of nursing procedures	Patient acceptability	Cost (£)
Foam replacement mattresses					
Performs better than a standard mattress — for medium risk patients	None required	Annual check for grounding	No problems	Generally good	90–160
Gel mattresses					
Suitable for medium to high risk patients	Heavy and difficult to move from one bed to another	None	May be difficult to move patients on it	Some patients may find the mattress unstable	500–800
Alternating pressure air mattresses					
Suitable for high risk patients	Some training needed; fairly simple to use	Annual maintenance check	Generally no problems	Mostly good; some find movement unpleasant	1500–3000
Airwave mattresses					
Suitable for high risk patients and those with pressure sores	Some training needed; fairly simple to use	Annual maintenance check	Generally no problems	Mostly good; some find it a little hard	3500
Dynamic air flotation mattresses					
Suitable for high risk patients and those with pressure sores	Some training needed; fairly simple to use	Annual maintenance check	Generally no problems	Mostly good; some find movement unpleasant	2750
Low air loss mattresses					
Suitable for high risk patients	Some training needed; fairly simple to use	Equipment most often rented	Generally no problems	Some find the pump noisy	rental

Table 5.2: Assessing overlays, mattresses and beds (contd)

Effectiveness	Ease of use	Maintenance	Ease of nursing procedures	Patient acceptability	Cost (£)
Low air loss beds					
Suitable for high risk patients and those with pressure sores	Complex equipment; training needed	Usually rented	Generally no problems; some may find the bed high	Generally good	Rental
Air-fluidised beds					
Suitable for high risk patients and those with pressure sores	Training needed	Usually rented	Generally no problems	Generally good	Rental

Table 5.2: Assessing overlays, mattresses and beds (contd)

Standard hospital mattress

The standard hospital mattress is still the most widely used mattress. It is made of a block of foam with edges of slightly denser foam. The standard cover is made from nylon coated with PVC to make it waterproof. It has an easily recognisable pink marble pattern. Some mattresses are supplied with a green Staphcheck cover which is intended to resist bacterial contamination. A more recent development is the Cromarty cover which is a one-way stretch material. Swain (1993) found that the Staphcheck cover caused hammocking and considerably higher interface pressures than the Cromarty cover which caused significantly lower pressures.

A number of problems with the standard mattress have been identified. The foam has a finite lifespan and will ultimately collapse so that it provides no support at all. The Department of Health recommends that mattresses should be expected to last for 4 years. Many hospitals, however, may have mattresses many years older than this. A mattress replacement programme should be established in all areas. Mattresses and beds supplied for community use are frequently cast-offs from hospitals. Regular mattress audit should be carried out in equipment stores as well as in hospitals.

Hospital mattresses have been shown to be a source of infection once the cover is no longer waterproof. The nylon covers lose their water resistance if sprayed with alcohol for cleansing. They should be cleaned with soap and water. The Staphcheck covers eventually crack and small pieces flake away from the cotton backing, leaving holes in the cover. Once moisture seeps into the foam, it provides fertile ground for bacterial growth. Three studies have highlighted the potential problems of infection. Fujita *et al* (1981) reported on an outbreak of infection in a burns unit caused by gentamicin-resistant *Pseudomonas aeruginosa*. Mattresses in the unit were found to be the source of the infection. Ten years later, Ndwula and Brown (1991) found mattresses to be the source of epidemic methicillin-resistant *Staphylococcus aureus* in an obstetric unit, which affected both mothers and babies and took 9 months to eradicate. In both cases the infection was resolved by replacing the contaminated mattresses. In a recent study, O'Donoghue and Allen (1992) calculated the cost of treating 10 orthopaedic patients with wound infection to be £22 200 compared with only £181.70 to replace the five defective mattresses which had carried the infection. *Figure 5.2* shows mould growing on a foam mattress and the 'tidemark' where it has been impregnated with moisture. Any mattress that is seen to have wet foam is a potential hazard and should be replaced immediately.

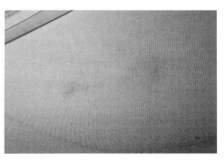

Swain (1993) suggested that the standard hospital mattress provides only minimum comfort and that it is not suitable for patients at risk of developing pressure sores. He also recommends that the Staph-check covers should no longer be used. The Cromarty cover would seem to be a better alter- native.

Figure 5-2: A foam mattress on which mould is growing

Overlays

Hollow core fibre overlays are widely used and many different brands are available. They look like a thick duvet, being divided into a series of cross segments or compartments. They provide both pressure reduction and comfort. They are particularly popular with frail, elderly patients who feel the cold as the material of the overlay provides extra warmth. A major drawback has been the problem of hospital laundry as the fibres become matted after they have been washed and then dried at too high a temperature. Increasingly, manufacturers are providing integral water-resistant, vapour-permeable, multi-stretch covers to over- come this problem.

Two studies have included a hollow core fibre overlay (Stapleton, 1986; Conine *et al*, 1990). Each study compared the overlay with large cell, alternating pressure air mattresses which had been found to be unreliable and to suffer frequent breakdown. Stapleton found no significant difference between the two. Overall, Conine *et al* found no significant difference in the total numbers of patients developing pressure sores. However, there were significantly higher numbers of sores on the trochanter in the overlay group. Furthermore, 59% of patients at high risk developed pressure sores while on the overlay. Hollow core fibre overlays are therefore probably best used for patients in the low risk category.

Another type of overlay which is increasing in popularity is the foam overlay. These overlays are usually 8–10 cm in depth and the surface is slashed to allow it to conform to body contours, thus reducing the interface pressure. A variety of water-resistant covers are available, some of which are two-way stretch which prevents hammocking. Swain (1994) compared a range of static overlays and found that the foam overlays gave good pressure reduction over all bony prominences. They can be used for low to medium risk patients.

Gel overlays are made of a thick gel which helps to disperse the pressure. The cover is washable. A review of the literature found only one study involving a gel overlay. Strunk and Osterbrunk (1988) studied patients undergoing cardiac surgery and compared the use of a gel overlay and a static air overlay with the standard foam on the operating table. They found that both the gel and the air overlay produced significantly lower interface pressures than the standard foam. Gel overlays are used to a limited extent on operating tables, but have not been used much on beds. They are rather heavy and cumbersome to use and may feel cold to the touch.

There are several types of air overlays. They all function slightly differently and so will be described separately. Static air overlays are made from PVC or rubber. They are constructed in such a way as to have cellular divisions. The patient is meant to sink into the overlay rather than lie on it. The overlays are inflated by means of a hand pump. Swain (1994) found that they gave good pressure reduction provided that they were inflated correctly. The amount of air required depends on the weight of the patient. Dealey (1995) suggested that this type of system may be better for single patient use rather than multiple use. Schregel *et al* (1993) compared a number of different support systems with the standard hospital mattress. They found that the static air overlays gave good pressure reduction of more than 50% compared with the standard mattress. The static air overlay is possibly suitable for medium to high risk patients, provided that it is correctly inflated.

There are two types of alternating pressure air overlay: the large cell and the small oval 'bubble pads'. Cells are alternately inflated and then deflated, the time cycle varying according to individual models. Some have removable covers made from two-way stretch, vapour-permeable materials which can be laundered. Some also have a transport facility whereby the patient can be moved on the bed without the overlay deflating. Several randomised controlled trials of alternating pressure air overlays have been carried out (Bliss, 1967; Anderson *et al*, 1982; Exton-Smith *et al*, 1982; Stapleton, 1986; Conine *et al*, 1990). These studies show that the system is significantly better than the standard hospital mattress, although the earlier versions were prone to breakdown. Newer versions are much more reliable and are suitable for medium to high risk patients.

The final overlay to be discussed is the low air loss overlay. This system is made of a permeable material divided into a number of cells. Air is constantly pumped into the overlay where it slowly passes out through the material. The patient sinks into and is supported by the overlay, which provides pressure reduction. Some patients may find the pump rather noisy. Some systems have a separate cover to aid laundry, although most of these systems are rented rather than purchased. A review of the literature found one study that included the low air loss bed (Thompson-Bishop and Molta, 1992). In this study interface pressures were recorded for healthy volunteers. The pressures recorded using the low air loss bed were considerably lower than those recorded using a standard hospital mattress.

In general, overlays can be useful support systems. It is immediately obvious when they are on a bed. They are mostly easy to use. Attention must be paid to the effect of raising the height of the bed, especially on fixed height beds. This may make the mobilisation and transfer of patients slightly more difficult.

Mattresses

Foam replacement mattresses have been introduced in some areas as an alternative to the standard hospital mattress. There are two main types: those made of different densities of foam and those with a slashed surface. Hofman *et al* (1994) compared a slashed foam mattress with a standard mattress for elderly patients with fractured neck of femur. They found that 25% and 68% respectively of patients developed pressure sores. However, Swain (1993) found that the mattresses made of foam of different densities lasted better in clinical use than the slashed foam models. Gray and

Campbell (1994) compared a replacement foam mattress with a standard mattress and found a significantly higher incidence of pressure sores with the standard mattress. Foam replacement mattresses are suitable for use by medium risk patients and are especially useful for orthopaedic and spinal cord injured patients.

Gel mattresses are made of foam with cells of gel which is slightly fluid and flows from one cell to another. These mattresses are heavy and therefore difficult to transfer from one bed frame to another. Some patients find it difficult to move on them as the gel cells make the mattress feel unstable. Lazzara and Buschmann (1991) compared a gel mattress with a static air overlay and found no significant difference between the two.

There is now available a variety of large cell, alternating pressure air mattresses which have two-way stretch covers and are a great improvement on the original alternating pressure systems. Research into their efficacy tends to consist of laboratory interface pressure measurements using healthy volunteers. Swain (1992) proposed a methodology which could be used in other centres and would allow comparison of results. This includes standardised positioning of sensors and frequency of measurements, and standardised positioning of elderly volunteers on the bed/mattress. These mattresses can be used for medium to high risk patients and for those with pressure sores.

Two more sophisticated examples of alternating pressure air mattresses have been developed: the Airwave system and the dynamic air flotation mattress. The Airwave system has a double layer of cells which work in groups of three so that one is inflated, one partially inflated and one deflated. The dynamic air flotation system has large cells which inflate alternately. It also has a sensor pad which allows automatic adjustment of pressure according to the weight of the patient. Exton Smith *et al* (1982) found the Airwave system to be much more reliable than the large cell ripple mattress. They also found that it was effective in pressure sore prevention. In a laboratory comparison of interface pressures, however, Swain *et al* (1992) found no difference in performance between these two sophisticated systems and suggested that a clinical trial was needed to evaluate their performance in pressure sore prevention. Subsequently, Devine (1995) compared the use of these two systems for patients with established pressure sores. He found that both systems were effective in the treatment of these patients. It can therefore be concluded that alternating pressure air mattresses are suitable for both high risk patients and those with pressure sores.

Low air loss mattresses work on the same principles as the overlay. Again, they tend to be rented rather than purchased because of their cost. The mattresses are more sophisticated than the overlays and may be adjusted for pressures, cycle time and temperature. Some have the ability to tilt the patient slightly from side to side. Thompson-Bishop and Mottola (1992) found that this type of mattress generated lower interface pressures than a standard hospital mattress.

Beds

The two types of beds currently available both provide pressure reduction. Low air loss beds are very sophisticated and expensive. As a consequence, they are often rented rather than purchased. The manufacturers have established a nurse advisor service to provide nurse and patient education and to monitor bed usage. These beds have a series of air sacs along their length which have a constant air flow that maintains pressures below 30 mmHg. The bed has electrical controls which allows the patient to be moved in the bed with greater ease. Some have built-in scales which can be very useful when monitoring patients with gross oedema or those with severe burns. In others, sacs in the central section of the bed may be deflated to assist mobilisation. Some beds at the top end of the range have the ability to rotate or oscillate to improve respiratory function. This is sometimes called kinetic therapy. Ferrell *et al* (1993) compared a kinetic low air loss bed with a foam overlay on a standard mattress for elderly patients with grade 2 pressure sores. They found a significantly faster healing rate among those patients on the low air loss bed.

This type of bed is quite high and some cannot be lowered, which causes difficulty in getting patients out of bed. However, they are of particular value for patients who show signs of pressure damage on other systems, for those who have to remain in one position, for heavy patients, for those who are difficult to move, and for those with severe pressure sores.

The air-fluidised bed consists of a large tank filled with ceramic particles. The motor causes air to flow through the particles to provide a flotation effect. The bed exerts pressures of about 11 mmHg. These beds are only available for rental and the manufacturers provide a nurse advisor service.

Allman *et al* (1987) compared air-fluidised beds with an alternating pressure air mattress for patients with pressure sores, and found a faster healing rate with the air-fluidised beds. Inman *et al* (1993) carried out a controlled clinical trial comparing an air-fluidised bed with a standard intensive care bed for patients in an intensive therapy unit. They found a higher incidence of pressure sores in the patients on the standard intensive care bed than in those on the air-fluidised bed.

Allman *et al* (1987) expressed reservations about air-fluidised beds in view of the difficulties in transferring patients on such beds. They are perhaps best used for patients who are confined to bed. They are especially useful for patients suffering from burns, major trauma or major surgery with heavily exuding wounds.

Selection of the low air loss and air -fluidised beds depends on clinical judgment. As these beds are very expensive, the decision should be based on informed clinical judgment.

Hospital guidelines can provide assistance in making appropriate decisions. Aronovitch (1992) made a retrospective study of their use to establish suitable criteria for selection. She found that health status, mental state, mobility, hydration, continence and nutrition were all relevant. A total of 26 patients had pressure sores, of whom nine were healed, 9 were improved and eight were worse at the end of the study. She concluded that assessment for risk factors was helpful in selection of this type of equipment.

Seating

There is a misconception that once patients are out of bed they are no longer at risk of developing pressure sores. This has resulted in patients sitting for long periods of time with no consideration of the need to relieve pressure. Gebhardt and Bliss (1994) compared the outcomes for two groups of elderly orthopaedic patients. One group sat out for unlimited periods and the other group sat out for no more than 2 hours at a time. They found a strong correlation between pressure sore development and the length of time spent sitting.

Dealey *et al* (1991) surveyed the chairs in an elderly care hospital and found that 77% either needed repair or had an obvious indentation in the cushion or a cushion with foam

5.3 Chair that provides very poor patient support

Figure 5.4: Chair that provides good patient support

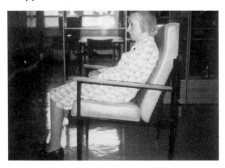
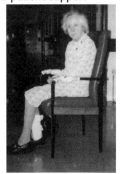

that was grounded; some had a combination of the three faults. It was also obvious that a number of the chairs maintained a very poor patient posture. *Figure 5.3* shows a patient in a chair with a backrest at about 30°. The patient is slumped in the chair and would not find it easy to rise to standing. In *Figure 5.4* the same patient is seated in a chair that provides much better support and much easier involvement in social activities. This study demonstrates the need to audit chairs as well as mattresses on a regular basis. Eden (1995) found that testing for grounding was a more accurate method of checking the pressure-reducing capacity of a chair than the visual check of cushion indentation.

Any type of seating is usually a compromise between comfort and function. Comfort includes pressure reduction. However, function is not only important in assisting in the maintenance of mobility and activity, but also ensures good posture. If a patient is seated in a good position there is less risk of shear and friction. *Figure 5.3* shows how the patient is at risk of sliding down in the chair.

Chairs

Many manufacturers claim that much effort has been invested into developing their chairs, with advice taken from occupational therapists. Unfortunately, there is little published evidence to support their claims. Dealey *et al* (1991) evaluated an armchair with a gel cushion. They found that it gave good support and pressure reduction. Patients were less likely to tip to one side. They noted the importance of having chairs at varying heights to aid patient mobility. They also found that the width of the arm was too wide for some patients to grasp. The chair has subsequently been modified and now has a wooden end on the arm. It must be remembered that many patients have to hold on to the chair to help them to rise to a standing position.

Some patients are unable to sit in conventional chairs

because of severe postural problems. Eden *et al* (1992) evaluated a chair specifically designed for this type of patient. They found it was excellent for confused or agitated patients and enabled seriously ill patients to sit out of bed for short periods. It was not suitable for any patient who is to be rehabilitated.

Cushions

There are a wide range of cushions available for use in wheelchairs. They are made of similar materials to the overlays and mattresses already discussed. They are an essential addition to the wheelchair. The wheelchair canvas exerts very high pressures. Dealey *et al* (1991) found pressures ranging from 120 mmHg to 200 mmHg. No one should remain seated on the wheelchair canvas for more than a very short time. Foam cushions 3 inches deep are most widely used and suitable for general use. Patients who are wheelchair-bound need to have a specialist assessment which is beyond the remit of this book. Advice can be obtained from the physiotherapist or occupational therapist. Coggrave *et al* (1994) described a seating clinic for subjects with spinal cord injury. They found it an effective method of providing appropriate seating for their patients.

Padding

There may be occasions when additional padding will be useful for protecting specific bony prominences. For example, if a patient has contractures of the legs, the knees may be held closely together, putting the patient at risk of pressure sore development at that point. The standard method of dealing with this is to place a pillow between the knees. However, with very rigid contractures this may not be possible. A small sheet of high density gel can be used. This has the effect of absorbing and spreading the pressure.

Additional padding may also be useful for the orthopaedic patient who has limited mobility. Such patients are often vulnerable to heel sores. Foam troughs are often used to lift the heel clear of the bed. Guin *et al* (1991) tested a number of devices that are used to reduce pressure over heels. They found that they all gave some pressure reduction, although some did not stay in position very well.

Pillows may also be used as a form of padding. They can be useful but consideration must be given to the quality of the pillow. If the cover is stiff plastic, it may cause sweating. The infill of the pillow may become lumpy over time, making the pillow uncomfortable to use.

Conclusions

There is a very wide range of equipment available for use, but more research is needed to determine the efficacy of much of the equipment that is in general use. Some hospitals are developing flow charts as part of their pressure sore prevention policy to assist in appropriate selection. The draft national *Clinical Practice Guidelines* (Collinson and Hitch, 1995) suggest some key points relating to equipment. These are listed below.

Key points

1. There should be a wide range of support systems available for use, which reflect the population at risk

2. Equipment should be tested, maintained and replaced on a regular basis

3. There should be audit of the usage and availability of

support systems

4. There should be a recognised procedure for obtaining equipment in all healthcare settings

5. Before purchasing equipment, the user should ask for information regarding its efficacy from the manufacturer

6. The equipment strategy should be reviewed in the light of any new research evidence

Based on Collinson and Hitch (1995)

References

Allman RM, Walker JM, Hart MK, Laprade CA, Noel LB, Smith CR (1987) Air-fluidised beds or conventional therapy for pressure sores. A randomised trial. *Ann Intern Med* **107**: 641–8

Anderson KE, Jenson O, Kvorning SA, Bach E (1982) Decubitus prophylaxis trial on the efficiency of alternating pressure air mattresses and water mattresses. *Acta Derm Venereol* **63**: 227–30

Aronovitch SA (1992) A retrospective study of the use of speciality beds in the medical and surgical intensive care units of a tertiary care facility. *Decubitus* **5**(1): 36–42

Bliss M (1967) Preventing pressure sores in hospital: controlled trial of a large celled ripple mattress. *Br Med J* **i**: 394–7

Bliss M, Thomas J (1992) Randomised controlled trials of pressure relieving supports. *J Tissue Viabil* **2**(3): 89–95

Clark M, Cullum N (1992) Matching patient need for pressure sore prevention with the supply of pressure redistributing mattresses. *J Adv Nurs* **17**: 310–16

Coggrave M, Rose L, Bogie K (1994) The role of a seating clinic in pressure sore prevention for spinal cord injured subjects. In: Harding KG, Dealey C, Cherry G, Gottrup F, eds. *Proceedings of the 3rd European Conference on Advances in*

Wound Management. Macmillan Magazines Ltd, London

Collinson G, Hitch S (1995) Prevention and Management of Pressure Sores: Clinical Practice Guidelines. Draft Guideline Synopsis. Conference on Clinical Effectiveness: From Guidelines to Cost-Effective Practice, May 3–4, London

Conine TA, Daechsel D, Laus MS (1990) The role of alternating air and silicore overlays in preventing decubitus ulcers. *Int J Rehabil Res* **15**: 133–7

Dealey C (1990) How are you supporting your patients? *Prof Nurse* **6**(3): 134–41

Dealey C (1991) The size of the pressure sore problem in a teaching hospital. *J Adv Nurs* **16**: 663–70

Dealey C (1992) Pressure sores: the result of bad nursing? *Br J Nurs* **1**(15): 748

Dealey C (1995) Mattresses and beds. *J Wound Care* **4**(9): 409–12

Dealey C, Earwaker T, Eden L (1991) Are your patients sitting comfortably? *J Tissue Viabil* **1**(2): 36–9

Devine B (1995) Alternating pressure air mattresses in the management of established pressure sores. *J Tissue Viabil* **5**(3): 94–8

Eden L (1995) *Testing armchairs*. Paper presented at Tissue Viability Society Conference, 28/29 March, Derby

Eden L, Earwaker T, Dealey C (1992) The management of patients with major seating difficulties. In: Harding Kg, Leaper DL, Turner TD, eds. *Proceedings of the 1st European Conference on Advances in Wound Care*. Macmillan Magazines, London

Effective Health Care Bulletin(1995) *The Prevention and Treatment of Pressure Sores, Vol 2(1)*. Nuffield Institute for Health, University of Leeds and NHS Centre for Reviews and Dissemination, University of York, published in association with Churchill Livingstone (copyright held by NHS Centre for Reviews and Dissemination and Nuffield Institute for Health

Exton Smith AN, Overstall PW, Wedgwood J, Wallace G (1982) The use of the 'Airwave System' to prevent pressure sores in hospital. *Lancet* **i**: 1288–90

Ferrell BA, Osterweil D, Christenson P (1993) A randomised trial of low air loss beds for treatment of pressure ulcers. *JAMA* **259(4)**: 494–7

Fujita K, Lilly HA, Kidson A, Ayliffe GAJ (1981) Gentamicin resistant *Pseudomonas aeruginosa* infection in a burns unit. *Br Med J* **283**: 219–20

Gebhardt K, Bliss M (1994) Preventing pressure sores in orthopaedic patients — is prolonged chair nursing detrimental? *J Tissue Viabil* **4**(2): 51–4

Gray D, Campbell M (1994) A randomised clinical trial of two types of foam mattress. *J Tissue Viabil* **4**(4): 128–32

Guin P, Hudson A, Gallo J (1991) The efficacy of six heel pressure reducing devices. *Decubitus* **4**(3): 15–23

Hibbs P (1990) The economics of pressure sore prevention. In: Bader D, ed. *Pressure Sores — Clinical Practice and Scientific Approach*. Macmillan Press, London: 35–42

Hitch S (1995) NHS Executive Nursing Directorate — strategy for major clinical guidelines — prevention and management of pressure sores: a review of the literature. *J Tissue Viabil* **5**(1): 3–24

Hofman A, Geelkerken RH, Wille J, Hamming JJ, Hermans J, Breslau PJ (1994) Pressure sores and pressure-decreasing mattresses: controlled clinical trial. *Lancet* **343**: 568–71

Inman KJ, Sibbald WJ, Rutledge FS, Clark BJ (1993) Clinical utility and cost-effectiveness of an air suspension bed in the prevention of pressure ulcers. *JAMA* **269**(9): 1139–43

Lazzara DJ, Buschmann MT (1991) Prevention of pressure ulcers in elderly nursing home residents: are special support services the answer? *Decubitus* **4**(4): 42–8

Ndwula EM, Brown L (1991) Mattresses as reservoirs of epidemic methicillin-resistant *Staphylococcus aureus*. *Lancet* **337**(8739): 488

O'Donoghue MAT, Allen KD (1992) Costs of an outbreak of wound infections in an orthopaedic ward. *J Hosp Infect* **22**: 73–9

Royal College of Physicians (1986) Disability in 1986 and beyond. *J R Coll Physicians Lond* **20**(3): 160–94

Schregal W, Hube M, Finsterwalder H (1993) Static and dynamic anti-decubitus systems for ITU care patients. *J Tissue Viabil* **3**(4): 108–13

Stapleton M (1986) Preventing pressure sores — an evaluation of three products. *Geriatr Nurs* March/April: 23–5

Strunk H, Osterbrunk K (1988) Pressure induced skin lesions in cardiac surgery. *Care Sci Pract* **6**(4): 113–15

Swain I (1992) Assessment of support surfaces. *Nurs Stand* **6**(Suppl 23): 12–14

Swain I (1993) *Evaluation: Foam Mattresses. A Comparative Evaluation*. Medical Devices Directorate. HMSO, London

Swain I (1994) *Evaluation: Static Mattress Overlays. A Comparative Evaluation*. Medical Devices Directorate. HMSO, London

Swain I, Nash R, Robertson J (1992) Assessment of support surfaces: comparison of Nimbus and Pegasus mattresses. *J Tissue Viabil* **2**(2): 43–5

Thompson-Bishop JY, Mottola CM (1992) Tissue interface pressure and estimated subcutaneous pressures of 11 different pressure-reducing support surfaces. *Decubitus* **5**(2): 42–8

Young J (1992a) Preventing pressure sores: does the mattress work? *J Tissue Viabil* **2**(1): 17

Young J (1992b) The use of specialised beds and mattresses. *J Tissue Viabil* **2**(3): 79–81

Chapter 6
The management of pressure sores

Introduction

The management of pressure sores can be quite complex. It is not just a case of putting a dressing on a wound. A thorough assessment of both the patient and the wound should be undertaken. Any factors that may delay healing should be identified and rectified where possible. A plan of care for managing the pressure sore should be instigated. Appropriate strategies to prevent further tissue damage should also be implemented. Accurate documentation will help to ensure continuity of care and aid evaluation of progress. Each of these issues will be discussed in further detail.

Patient assessment

The assessment and management of any wound should include assessment of the patient. A number of factors can delay healing. If they go unrecognised and untreated the patient will continue to suffer — often unnecessarily. Dealey (1994) considers that physical, psychological and spiritual aspects should be addressed. It should also be noted that some of the factors that delay healing may have contributed to the pressure damage in the first instance.

Physical assessment

The activities of daily living (Roper *et al*, 1990) make a useful framework for a physical assessment.

Maintaining a safe environment

One aspect of maintaining a safe environment is consideration of infection and infection control. If the wound is infected it will not heal or may start to heal and break down again. Infection elsewhere, such as in the chest or urinary tract use the same resources that are needed to heal a wound. Consequently, wound healing may be delayed. Simple measures such as good handwashing techniques are therefore essential (Gould, 1992).

Another aspect of maintaining a safe environment is to prevent the development of further pressure sores or the deterioration of existing sores. Obviously, the patient will still be at risk of further pressure sore development and will need to be monitored carefully.

Communicating

Nursing is often described as an art as well as a science. One aspect of the art of nursing is the ability to communicate with patients. This involves listening effectively to what is spoken and unspoken, and recognising the anxieties that many patients have about a whole host of issues.

Stress and anxiety have physiological effects as well as emotional effects. As well as an increase in adrenaline release, there is an increase in adrenocorticotrophic hormone release which stimulates the adrenal cortex to produce increased amounts of glucocorticoids; these break down tissue to provide extra energy in the form of glucose. The immune system is suppressed and there is a reduced inflammatory response. Increased breakdown of protein results in delayed collagen production, all of which delay healing.

A variety of factors can act as stressors and produce this physiological effect. Physical stressors include trauma, surgery and pain. Pain can not only be increased by anxiety, but can itself increase anxiety. Unrelieved pain may reduce mobility: if it hurts a patient to move, then he/she is more likely to keep still. Whereas many patients with deep pressure sores seem to suffer amazingly little pain, those with more superficial sores may find them very painful. Patients should always be assessed for pain. If they have persistent pain, the use of an objective assessment tool, such as a pain ruler (Bourbonnais, 1981), will assist in evaluating the effectiveness of pain control.

Breathing

Oxygen is essential for healing, and so a good blood supply is needed. This is a situation where factors that could have been relevant to pressure damage will also delay healing. For example, with advancing age the general circulation may be less efficient. There is also an increased risk of disease, such as peripheral vascular disease which can result in poor tissue perfusion.

Eating and drinking

Malnutrition is a pathological state that results from a deficiency of one or more essential nutrients. It has been associated with pressure sore development (see Chapter 2). It will also affect the healing process as carbohydrates, protein, fats, vitamins A, B and C and minerals such as zinc are all required. The identification of patients who are susceptible to malnutrition was discussed in Chapter 4.

Eliminating

Incontinence has been associated with pressure sore development. In addition, a wound that is constantly contaminated with urine and faeces is very difficult to manage.

Patients with uraemia experience difficulties in wound healing, although the mechanism for this is not clearly understood. A blood urea above 7 mmol/litre will delay both granulation and epithelialisation (Barton and Barton, 1981).

Personal cleansing and dressing

Poor standards of hygiene increase the risk of bacterial contamination and, potentially, wound infection. Many patients 'fiddle' with their wounds, especially confused patients.

Maintaining body temperature

Persistent pyrexia increases the metabolic rate, thereby increasing nutritional requirements. Each degree rise in body temperature increases energy expenditure by 10% (Goode *et al*, 1985), yet pyrexia may also be associated with a loss of appetite and dehydration. Pyrexia may be an indicator of infection and should not be ignored.

Mobilising

It is important to recognise the effects of poor mobility as well as identifying its causes. Prolonged sitting will result in stasis oedema in the lower limbs. Pressure sores in this area may be slow in healing because of the sluggish blood supply. Mobility may be reduced for only a short period of time, eg. in the postoperative period. It can also be associated with disease, such as rheumatoid disease. This is an inflammatory disease and is often treated with anti-inflammatory drugs. When these drugs are used for long periods of time they can have an inhibitory effect on the healing of chronic wounds such as pressure sores (Lawrence and Payne, 1984).

Expressing sexuality

Sexuality and body image are closely linked to self-esteem. A wound can cause alterations in body image which can affect a person's view of him/herself. While pressure sores generally develop on parts of the body that are not commonly on view and so are not likely to affect body image, they may not be the only wounds with which a patient has to come to terms. Disfiguring wounds of the face, mastectomy or amputation may all cause great distress to the patient. Equally, an offensive, heavily exuding pressure sore can cause distress. Any of these can act as stressors, the physiological effects of which have already been discussed.

Sleeping

It is well known that many people experience difficulty in sleeping while in hospital: there are often disturbances in the ward; most people are not used to sleeping in a room with a number of other people; the bed may be uncomfortable; or the patient may be in pain. The need for a good night's sleep is often dismissed and yet everyone is familiar with the sense of wellbeing that it imparts. Florence Nightingale (1859) emphasised the importance of sleep in aiding recovery from illness. Adam and Oswald (1984) suggested that sleep helped to promote tissue repair as there is increased release of somatotrophin, testosterone and prolactin during sleep.

Dying

A dying patient may not have the ability to heal his/her wounds, possibly because there is not enough time left to the patient to heal a large wound or because the disease process is affecting the ability of the wound to heal. This can be very distressing to the nurse, especially if further pressure damage occurs despite intensive preventive measures. In the end stage of some diseases the peripheral blood supply may be compromised, and even very little pressure may result in damage to the skin. While every effort should be made to prevent this occurring, prevention is not always possible. It is essential to identify patient problems rather than nursing problems and address these. An example might be distress at dressing change: in this situation the frequency of dressing change should be reduced as much as possible. The main goal should always be to allow the patient to die with dignity.

Psychological assessment

A number of psychological problems may act as stressors. Some of the common ones are fear, grief and powerlessness or a loss of control over one's life or environment. Many patients may suffer one or more of these stressors and react in a variety of ways. Some become quiet and withdrawn, whereas others may be angry or aggressive. The nurse is often the first person to recognise the signs of psychological distress. Further help may be needed. Advice can be sought from a clinical psychologist, chaplain, psychiatric nurse or a trained counsellor.

Spiritual assessment

While there has been an improvement in nurses' understanding of the psychological needs of individual patients, there is less recognition of spiritual needs. Spirituality is a wider concept than identifying an individual's religious persuasion. Fish and Shelley (1985) defined spiritual needs as the need for meaning and purpose, the need for love and relatedness and the need for forgiveness. Spiritual pain or distress results if these needs are not met. Morrison (1992) suggests that spiritual pain is the result of loss of meaning due to the shattering of a person's view of life.

Further exploration of the concept of meaning and purpose may help to explain this. Each person gains meaning and purpose in life by the roles he/she fulfils. For example, a nurse may also be a child, a parent, a husband or wife, a member of a society and so on. If a person is unable to fulfil these roles for any length of time, spiritual distress will follow. A dramatic example is a person involved in an accident that renders him/her paraplegic or tetraplegic. That person would have to work through considerable pain to come to terms with loss of much of his/her previous purpose in life and develop new roles. Obviously, such distress acts as a stressor, the physiological effects of which have already been discussed.

Pressure sore assessment

Assessment of the patient provides much useful information. Assessment of the wound should include:

- Pressure sore grading
- Assessment of the wound bed
- Exudate levels
- Position of the sore
- Assessment of the wound margins

Pressure sore grading

The use of a system for grading pressure sores is an attempt to identify the severity of the sore, usually by indicating the depth of tissue damage. It can be a useful measurement, but the method used needs to be understood by all who are caring for the patient or reading any report involving pressure sores. There is a whole host of grading systems from which to choose. Hitch (1995) identified 10 different systems for grading pressure sores in her review of the literature. Obviously, there is some variation between them; however, the common feature is that the higher the grade the deeper the sore. Gradings may range from 0 to 7, but the most common range is 1 to 4 or 5.

Some grading systems start with persistent blanching erythema. This indicates an area of redness that blanches under light fingertip pressure. There has been a certain amount of debate over this criterion. Lyder (1991) discussed the concept of the stage 1 pressure sore and proposed a number of criteria for which, he argued, there was scientific evidence to support their inclusion. They are listed in *Table 6.1*. Both the national Clinical Practice Guidelines for Pressure Sore Prevention and Management (Collinson and Hitch, 1995) and the *American Clinical Practice Guideline: Pressure Ulcers in Adults: Prediction and Prevention* (Agency for Health Care Policy and Research, 1992) support the use of non-blanching erythema as the definition of a grade 1 pressure sore.

Table 6.1: Criteria for stage 1 pressure sores

- A reddened area which ranges from pink to bright red

- A reddened area which does not blanch under light finger-tip pressure

- The skin area is warmer to the touch than surrounding skin

- A reddened area which does not fade within 2 hours

- Oedema and induration are present around the affected area

- The epidermis is still intact over the affected area

Based on Lyder, (1991)

Even when the concept of the grade 1 sore is clarified, there are still other difficulties in pressure sore grading to resolve. If the pressure sore is covered in a thick necrotic eschar, it is impossible to judge accurately the degree of tissue damage. It would certainly be greater than that of a grade 1 sore. Assessment of a pressure sore such as this is best delayed until the necrotic tissue has been debrided.

Assessment of pressure sores on patients with dark skin is also difficult as it may not be possible to see any reddened areas. Thus, considerable tissue damage may occur before it is noticed. While both of the guidelines mentioned above emphasises the need to ensure effective identification of grade 1 sores in those with a dark skin, neither suggests how it might be achieved. Anecdotal evidence suggests that the skin becomes dry and cracked over areas where erythema is present. However, further work is needed in this area to provide clear guidance.

One of the simpler grading systems is that used by David *et al* (1983) and sometimes called the Surrey Grading System. It is described below and illustrated in *Figure 6.1*.

Grade 1: Non-blanching erythema

Grade 2: Superficial break in the skin

Grade 3: Destruction of the skin without cavity

Grade 4: Destruction of the skin with cavity

The most recently published grading system is the Stirling Pressure Sore Severity Scale (Reid and Morison, 1994). This has grades from 0 to 4. Grade 0 indicates no evidence of a pressure sore. The remaining grades are basically the same as those cited above but each grade has a number of subsections. Each subsection is given a digit. Thus, the first two digits relate to the level and nature of tissue damage, the third digit describes the wound bed and the fourth digit codes for infection. An example of this grading in usage is a sore that is coded as grade 3.431, which means a pressure sore with full-thickness skin loss that is full of soft cream/ yellow/green slough and surrounded by inflammation. This system may be rather more accurate than other grading systems, but is likely to require considerable training to ensure that it is used accurately.

A recent study has considered the reliability and utility of three grading systems (Healey, 1995). One hundred and nine nurses were shown a series of 10 photographs and asked to grade the pressure sores according to three grading systems: Surrey, Stirling and Torrance (a five-grade system). Stat-

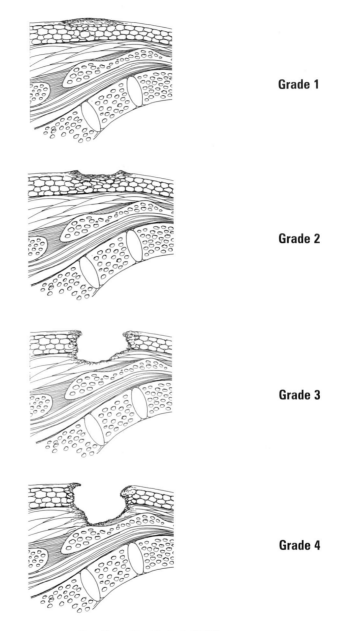

Figure 6.1: Pressure sore grading (from David *et al*, 1983)

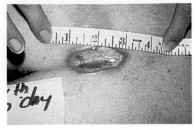

Figure 6.2:
A necrotic pressure
sore (probably grade 3)

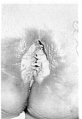

Figure 6.3:
An infected grade 4
pressure sore

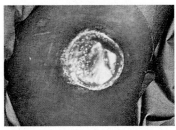

Figure 6.4:
A sloughy grade 3
pressure sore

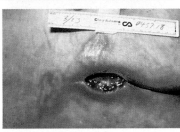

Figure 6.5:
A granulating grade 3
pressure sore

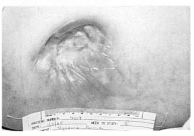

Figure 6.6:
An epitheliasing
grade 2 pressure sore

istical analysis of the results showed that there was a significantly lower interrater reliability for the Stirling score (39%) than for the other two grading systems (Torrance 60% and Surrey 69%). A significantly higher number of nurses found the Surrey score easiest to use, suggesting that the simpler the scoring system the greater the likelihood that it will be used effectively.

Assessment of the wound bed

Assessment of the wound bed will provide information about the wound appearance and exudate. This is very important when selecting suitable wound management products. Wound appearance can be divided into:

- Necrotic
- Infected
- Sloughy
- Granulating
- Epithelialising

Figures 6.2–6.6 p88 show examples of each type of wound.

Necrotic wounds

Following a period of ischaemia, the damaged tissue may form a necrotic eschar or scab which is usually black or brown. Necrotic tissue may also take the form of a thick grey slough. It should be recognised that necrotic tissue masks the extent of tissue damage. The pressure sore is likely to appear to have enlarged once the necrotic eschar has been removed.

Infected wounds

If a wound is infected it will not heal. However, the identification of infected chronic wounds is not always easy. Cutting and Harding (1994) discussed this problem and proposed some criteria for identifying infection in open wounds, in addition to the traditional criteria of swelling, heat, pain, redness and purulent discharge. The additional criteria are listed in *Table 6.2*. Cutting and Harding cited these criteria for use with all types of open wounds, but only their usefulness for assessing pressure sores will be considered here.

Table 6.2: Additional criteria for identifying infection in open wounds

1.	Delayed healing (compared with normal rate for site/condition)
2.	Discoloration
3.	Friable granulation tissue which bleeds easily
4.	Unexpected pain/tenderness
5.	Pocketing at the base of the wound
6.	Bridging at the base of the wound
7.	Abnormal smell
8.	Wound breakdown

From Cutting and Harding (1994)

Delayed healing: Unlike surgical wounds, there are no guidelines for healing rates of chronic wounds. Many other factors can delay healing. However, if a patient has several pressure sores, all of which are healing except one, then infection should be considered as a potential cause of delayed healing.

Discoloration: Infected wounds have an unhealthy appearance. Depending on the type of bacteria causing the infection, the wound bed may be a dull dark red or have patches of green/yellow discoloration.

Friable granulation tissue: Another indication of infection is granulation tissue which bleeds easily and has a red, raw appearance.

Unexpected pain/tenderness: This may be localised pain or a wound that is painful when touched.

Pocketing or bridging in the wound: This is more commonly found in surgical wounds.

Odour: Infected wounds may have an offensive odour. However, necrotic tissue can also have an extremely offensive odour.

Wound breakdown: Again, this is more commonly observed in a surgical wound, but can occur in pressure sores.

Sloughy wounds

Slough has a white/yellow colour and may be found in patches on the wound surface. In a moist environment, macrophages will gradually clear slough by phagocytosis. Slough may be present in small quantities even when a wound is healing and reducing in size. As long as the sore continues to make progress, the presence of slough should not cause any anxiety.

Granulating wounds

Once any necrotic tissue and general cell debris have been removed from the sore, there should be signs of granulation tissue. This is usually bright red with a granular or nobbly appearance.

Epithelialising wounds

Once any cavity has filled with granulation tissue, new epithelial cells will start to develop around the wound margins. They are a pinkish/white colour and will gradually migrate across the wound surface.

Exudate levels

The amount of exudate will vary and should be recorded. The terms most frequently used are high, moderate and low. Copious exudate may be an indication of infection, but can also be found during the autolysis of necrotic tissue. The degree of exudate from a wound will affect dressing selection.

Position of the sore

Recording the position of pressure sores has several benefits. The position can aid identification of the cause of a pressure sore. For example, a pressure sore over the ischial tuberosities may occur as a result of the patient sitting for long periods on an unsuitable surface. However, a sore on only one ischial tuberosity may be caused by the patient sitting tilted to one side. In both instances, not only the length of time a patient sits out but also the support surface need to be considered; in the latter case, however, improved postural support is also needed.

The position of the sore may affect dressing selection. Very often two or three different dressings may be suitable for the type of wound, but only one of them may be appropriate for the position of the sore. For example, retention of dressings over the sacrum is notoriously difficult. If a patient with a heel sore is being rehabilitated, then a non-bulky dressing may be most suitable when the patient is walking.

Regular recording of the position of pressure sores can be of benefit when monitoring pressure sores over a period of time. If a particular group of patients shows a high incidence of sores at a particular site, the cause may be an item of equipment or a specific procedure.

Assessment of the wound margins

Insufficient notice is usually taken of the skin around a pressure sore. Redness may indicate that there is further damage and that the sore is likely to extend. It may also indicate inadequate pressure relief over the site of the pressure sore. The surrounding skin may be fragile and vulnerable to superficial skin tears, particularly from adhesive tape. There may even be an indication of trauma from the frequent removal of adhesive tape. On the other hand, the surrounding skin may be firm and healthy, providing further evidence that the pressure sore is healing and that further breakdown is unlikely.

Documentation

Good record keeping provides accurate evidence of the progress, or otherwise, of a wound. This should include some form of measurement as well as a progress chart. Measurement may be a simple measurement of the dimensions of the sore or a tracing of the circumference. Some nurses have access to a camera which will provide an indication of wound appearance as well as size.

The Wound Care Society has produced a form for initial assessment (*Figure 6.7*) and an ongoing assessment sheet (*Figure 6.8*) (Flanagan, 1994). This type of assessment form should allow easy identification of any potential problems and can be readily adapted to most environments.

Pressure sore management

Pressure sore management is a combination of the ident-ification of factors that may delay healing and addressing them where possible, and appropriate dressing selection and implementation of prevention strategies to prevent further tissue damage.

Figure 6-7: Initial assessment chart

Wound Care Society assessment chart

Initial assessment

Names

| Patient name | Age |

| GP name |

Describe the wound

| Type of wound |

| Location of wound |

Wound dimensions

Max length [   ] cm/mm (delete as appropriate)

Max width [   ] cm/mm (delete as appropriate)

Depth [   ] cm/mm (delete as appropriate)

Length of time wound present [   ] days/weeks/months/years (delete as appropriate)

Risk assessment

Pressure sore risk assessment scale used [   ] Score [   ]

Doppler reading = Ankle pressure / Arm pressure [   ] mm/Hg Index [   ]

Condition of skin [ ] Good/intact [ ] Fair/red areas* [ ] Poor/breaks*

*Describe in more detail together with action taken

| |

Factors that may delay healing

Diabetes [ ]   Medications [ ]

Anaemia [ ]   Allergies [ ]

Immobility [ ]   Non-compliance [ ]

Poor nutritional status [ ]   Others [ ]

Referral requested Date

Clinical nurse specialist [   ]

Dermatologist [   ]

Vascular surgeon [   ]

Dietitian [   ]

Chiropodist [   ]

Others [   ]

Figure 6-8: Ongoing assessment chart

Date of dressing change										
Wound dimensions										
Max length (cm/mm)										
Max width (cm/mm)										
Depth (cm/mm)										
Are dimensions...										
Increasing?										
Decreasing?										
Static?										
Wound bed (approx % cover										
Necrotic (black(										
Slough (yellow)										
Granulating (red)										
Epithelialising (pink)										
Exudate levels										
High*										
Moderate										
Low										
Amount increasing*										
Amount decreasing										
*May indicate wound infection										
Wound margin/surrounding skin										
Macerated*										
Oedematous										
Erythema*										
Eczema										
Fragile*										
Dry/scaling										
Healthy/intact										
*May indicate wound infection										
Pain*										
Continuous										
At specific times										
At dressing change										
None										
*May indicate wound infection										
In addition, suspect wound infection if...										
Granulation tissue bleeds easily										
Fragile bridging of epithelium occurs										
Odour increases										
Healing is slower than anticipated										
Wound breakdown										
Action taken										
Swab sent										
Results obtained										
Treatment objective(s)										
Debridement										
Absorption										
Hydration										
Protection										
Documentation (7-10 day intervals) - tick when done										
Trace wound circumference										
Photograph										
Evaluate pressure risk-assessment score										
Signature/initial										

Factors that may delay healing

Accurate patient assessment will have identified any factors that may delay healing. The management plan should include the development of appropriate strategies to address those issues which can be resolved. For example, poor nutritional status can generally be improved, whereas increasing age cannot.

Appropriate dressing selection

This is a huge topic and can only be dealt with superficially here. The different categories of dressings and any evidence to support their use in pressure sore treatment will be discussed. Further reading on the topic is suggested at the end of this chapter.

There is a wide range of wound management products from which to choose. Selection should be based on assessment of the sore and the setting of relevant objectives. For example, a dressing that is appropriate for a grade 4 pressure sore with slough and a heavy exudate is not likely to be suitable for a grade 2 sore with little exudate.

Alginates

Alginate dressings are made from calcium and sodium alginate. The precise constituents vary according to the individual products. They are presented as a flat fibrous sheet or a fibrous rope of varying length and thickness. The alginate dressing absorbs exudate and forms a gel on the wound surface, thus maintaining a moist environment. Without exudate the dressing cannot gel. It is not, therefore, suitable for wounds with a low to moderate exudate. The rope dressing can be used in cavity wounds. Alginates can be used on all types of wounds with a moderate to heavy exudate. They can be used on infected wounds in conjunction with systemic antibiotics, but should be changed daily.

Meaume *et al* (1996) carried out a multi-centre

randomised controlled trial comparing an alginate with a bead dressing for cavity pressure sores. The alginate dressing was found to have a significantly faster healing rate and to be more cost-effective than the bead dressing.

Beads

Bead dressings are made from hydrophilic beads which swell and gel as they absorb exudate. Some contain soluble iodine. These dressings are best suited to infected or sloughy wounds with a copious exudate. When a bead dressing containing iodine is used, the manufacturers' instructions should be followed carefully as iodine can be absorbed systemically. Bead dressings have been compared with hydrogels and with alginates in the management of pressure sores. Two studies compared a bead dressing with a hydrogel dressing (Thomas and Fear, 1993; Colin *et al*, 1996). In both studies, the bead dressing took longer to debride sloughy wounds than the hydrogel.

Charcoals

Charcoal dressings have activated charcoal incorporated in their structure. This is able to absorb odour and is most useful for the management of malodorous wounds. Some forms of charcoal dressing comprise a sheet of activated charcoal and an absorbent pad, whereas others may be a combination dressing such as a combination foam and charcoal dressing. Charcoal dressings are generally used in conjunction with another dressing.

Enzymatic

This preparation contains two enzymes, streptokinase and streptodornase. It is presented as a powder and has to be reconstituted with sterile water or saline before use. It is intended for use on dry necrotic eschar. However, patients who have been treated with this product have shown an increase in serum antistreptokinase titres (Green, 1993).

Thus, it should only be used for those patients not at risk of myocardial infarction.

Films

Film dressings are made from semipermeable polyurethane adhesive film. They have varying methods of application depending on the product. They have no absorbency and are therefore suitable for clean wounds with low or no exudate. Banks *et al* (1994a) compared a film dressing combined with a low-adherent dressing with an adhesive foam dressing in the management of patients with grade 1 or 2 pressure sores. No difference in efficacy was found between the treatment regimens.

Foams

Foam dressings consist of varying presentations of polyurethane foam. Some are presented as a flat sheet with or without an adhesive backing. Others are presented as fillers for cavity wounds. Foam dressings absorb exudate and allow water vapour to pass out through the back of the dressing. They have varying absorbency depending on the product. They can be used on granulating and epithelialising wounds and on wounds with patchy slough. Banks *et al* (1994b) compared a thin adhesive foam dressing with a hydrocolloid for the treatment of shallow pressure sores. There was no difference in healing rates or frequency of dressing change, but the foam dressing was significantly easier to remove than the hydrocolloid.

Hydrocolloids

Hydrocolloid dressings are made from a polyurethane foam bonded to an adhesive mass. The latter is constructed from varying ingredients, including cellulose and pectin. The adhesive mass absorbs exudate, and then swells to form a gel. The outer side of the dressing is waterproof. Hydrocolloid pastes and powders are available for use in conjunction with a hydrocolloid sheet for small cavity wounds. They have varying absorbency but are generally best suited to wounds with a moderate to low exudate.

Several of the studies mentioned in this section use hydrocolloid dressings as the comparison dressing when evaluating a newer product. Hydrocolloids are well established as effective dressings for chronic wounds such as pressure sores (Dobrzanski *et al*, 1990) and are widely used, especially on grade 1–3 sores.

Hydrogels

Hydrogel dressings contain 70–96% water depending on the product. They are available as either a flat gel sheet or an amorphous gel. The amorphous gel may be used on both shallow wounds and small cavities and sinuses of all types. The gel sheets should be used for shallow granulating or epithelialising wounds. Neither presentation is suitable for wounds with a heavy exudate. As noted previously, hydrogel dressings debride sloughy pressure sores faster than do bead dressings. Flanagan (1995) measured the reduction in slough in 55 wounds using hydrogels. A consistent reduction in devitalised tissue by hydrogels was found during the study period.

Hydropolymers

This type of dressing is made from a mixture of polymers. They are hydrophilic but do not liquefy or breakdown. Banks *et al* (1996) compared a hydropolymer dressing with a hydrocolloid dressing for the treatment of grade 2 and 3 pressure sores. They found that both dressings performed equally well.

Prevention strategies

The prevention strategies and the use of pressure relieving equipment described in Chapters 4 and 5 are also suitable for use with patients with pressure sores.

Conclusion

Effective pressure sore management requires a holistic approach to assessment which will guide the development of appropriate management strategies.

Key points

1. Patient assessment should include physical, psychological and spiritual assessment

2. A pressure sore grading system should be used as part of the assessment process

3. Pressure sore assessment should include assessment of the wound bed, exudate levels, position of the sore and assessment of the wound margins, in addition to pressure sore grading

4. Accurate documentation assists in monitoring the progress of the pressure sore

5. Pressure sore management involves: addressing any factors that delay healing, appropriate wound management and implementation of prevention strategies

Further reading

Dealey C (1994) *The Care of Wounds: A Guide for Nurses*. Blackwell Scientific Publications, Oxford

References

Adam K, Oswald I (1984) Sleep helps healing. *Br Med J* **289**: 1400–1

Banks V, Bale S, Harding KG (1994a) Superficial pressure sores: comparing two regimes. *J Wound Care* **3**(1): 8–10

Banks V, Bale S, Harding KG (1994b) The use of two dressings for moderately exuding pressure sores. *J Wound Care* **3**(3): 132–4

Banks V, Fear M, Orphin J *et al* (1996) A comparative open multi-centre trial of Tielle hydropolymer dressing and granuflex improved formulation. In: Cherry GW, Gottrup F, Lawrence JC, Moffatt CJ, Turner TD, eds. *Proceedings of the 5th European Conference on Advances in Wound Management*. Macmillan Magazine, London: 163–7

Barton A, Barton M (1981) *The Management and Prevention of Pressure Sores*. Faber and Faber, London

Bourbonnais F (1981) Pain assessment: development of a tool for the nurse and patient. *J Adv Nurs* **6**(4): 277–82

Colin D, Kurring PA, Quinlan D, Yvon C (1996) The clinical investigation of an amorphous hydrogel compared with a dextranomer paste dressing in the management of sloughy wounds. In: Cherry GW, Gottrup F, Lawrence JC, Moffatt CJ, Turner TD, eds. *Proceedings of the 5th European Conference on Advances in Wound Management*. Macmillan Magazines, London: 155–9

Collinson G, Hitch S (1995) Pressure Sore Prevention and Management: Clinical Practice Guidelines. Guideline Synopsis. Conference on Clinical Effectiveness from Guidelines to Cost-Effective Practice, May 3–4, London

Cutting K, Harding KG (1994) Criteria for identifying wound

infection. *J Wound Care* **3**(4): 198–201

David J, Chapman RG, Chapman EG, Lockett B (1983) *An Investigation of the Current Methods used in Nursing for the Care of Patients with Established Pressure Sores.* Nursing Practice Research Unit, Northwick Park, Middx

Dealey C (1994) *The Care of Wounds: A Guide for Nurses.* Blackwell Scientific Publications, Oxford

Dobrzanski S, Kelly CM, Gray JI, Gregg AJ, Cosgrove CA (1990) Granuflex dressings in treatment of full thickness pressure sores. *Prof Nurse* **5**(11): 594–9

Fish S, Shelley JA (1985) *Spiritual Care: The Nurse's Role.* InterVarsity Press, Downers Grove, Illinois

Flanagan M (1994) Assessment criteria. *Nurs Times* **90**(35): 76–88

Flanagan M (1995) The efficacy of a hydrogel in the treatment of wounds with non-viable tissue. *J Wound Care* **4**(6): 264–7

Goode AW, Howard JP, Woods S (1985) *Clinical Nutrition and Dietetics for Nurses.* Hodder and Stoughton, London

Gould D (1992) Hygienic hand decontamination. *Nurs Stand* **6**(32): 33–6

Green C (1993) Antistreptokinase titres after topical streptokinase. *Lancet* **341**: 1602–3

Healey F (1995) The reliability and utility of pressure sore grading scales. *J Tissue Viabil* **5**(4): 111–14

Hitch S (1995) NHS Executive Nursing Directorate — strategy for major Clinical guidelines — prevention and management of pressures sores, a literature review. *J Tissue Viabil* **5**(1): 3–24

Lawrence JC, Payne HJ (1984) *Wound Healing.* The Update Group, London

Lyder CH (1991) Conceptualization of the stage 1 pressure sore. *J Enterostomal Ther Nurs* **18**(5): 162–5

Meaume S, Sayag J, Bonnefoy M et al (1996) Calcium alginate dressing (Algosteril ™) in the management of full-thickness pressure sores: a controlled, randomized study on elderly patients. In: Cherry GW, Gottrup F, Lawrence JC, Moffatt CJ, Turner TD, eds. *Proceedings of the 5th European Conference* on *Advances in Wound Management*. Macmillan Magazines, London: 19

Morrison R (1992) Diagnosing spiritual pain in patients. *Nurs Stand* **6**(25): 36–8

Nightingale F (1859) (Reprinted 1974) *Notes on Nursing: What it is and What it is Not*. Blackie and Son, Glasgow and London

Panel for the Prediction and Prevention of Pressure Ulcers in Adults (1992) Pressure ulcers in adults: Prediction and Prevention. AHCPR Publication, US Department of Health and Human Services, Rockville, Maryland

Reid J, Morison M (1994) Towards a consensus: classification of pressure sores. *J Wound Care* **3**(3): 157–60

Roper N, Logan W, Tierney A (1990) *The Elements of Nursing*. 3rd edn. Churchill Livingstone, Edinburgh

Thomas S, Fear M (1993) Comparing two dressings for wound depridement. *J Wound Care* **2**(5): 272–4

Chapter 7

Pressure sore prevention policies

Introduction

Since 1986 when the Royal College of Physicians called for each health district to have a written pressure sore prevention policy, there has been increasing interest in the subject (Royal College of Physicians, 1986). In 1987 the King's Fund Pressure Sore Group was formed and held several symposia to discuss the need for prevention strategies. The group published a booklet in 1989 to assist hospitals and health authorities in establishing a prevention policy. An updated version was published in 1993 (Simpson and Livesley, 1993). The guidance in this booklet provides the framework for this chapter.

Developing a policy

Simpson and Livesley (1993) describe five steps for developing a policy. They are:

1. Establish a pressure sore group

2. Collect baseline data about patients, resources and existing knowledge base of the staff

3. Identify problems and/or issues

4.   Develop and implement the policy

5.   Audit the effect.

Each of these steps will now be considered in detail.

The pressure sore group

It has already been established that pressure sore prevention requires a multidisciplinary approach. It is logical that the pressure sore group should be multidisciplinary in its membership. There should be representatives from nursing, medicine, pharmacy, physiotherapy, occupational therapy, dietetics and administration and/or facilities. In some trusts it may also be appropriate to include the ambulance service.

When establishing such a group it is very easy to end up with a large unwieldy group which will not be effective. All the members should be committed to the project and have respect for each other's clinical expertise. The ideal size for an effective group is about six to eight people. If the group has to be larger, it may be appropriate to divide it into a number of subgroups, each with specific tasks to carry out.

The chairperson should not be selected from political expediency, but because he/she is the best person for the job. It is obviously helpful if the chairperson has experience in organising disparate groups. In many areas, the clinical nurse specialist in tissue viability is the ideal person for this position because he/she is a recognised expert in the field and is able to give time to the project.

It is very easy for a project team to start with great enthusiasm and then lose its way. It is helpful for the group to set short- and long-term goals. It is also useful to have a formal framework for the meetings with an agenda and minutes. The minutes can be circulated to senior management to keep them informed of the progress of the project. Monthly meetings with a set time limit, such as one hour, are usually sufficient and do not put an undue burden on the group members.

Collect baseline data

Before starting to change any practice, it is important to determine current practice. The first task for the group to undertake is to obtain baseline information about the patients, resources and the level of knowledge of the clinical staff.

The patient population

Baseline data about the patient population are best obtained by means of a point prevalence survey. This can provide a whole host of information, depending on the questions that are asked. Dealey (1991) suggested that as well as identifying those patients with pressure sores, all patients should be assessed for their degree of risk. This gives some indication of the dependency of the patients and can be invaluable when planning equipment requirements.

Further information that could be obtained includes the position and grade of the pressure sores, and whether they developed in the current place of care, eg. a hospital, or were present on admission and/or transfer. Knowledge of the dressing regimen and the use of pressure-relieving equipment can also provide invaluable information about current practice.

When planning a prevalence survey, it is helpful to consider which risk calculator and pressure sore grading system are best suited to the patient population. Staff training will be required before the survey is carried out. Future confusion can be avoided if agreement can be reached regarding long-term methods of risk assessment and grading systems so that the methods used for the survey will continue in use afterwards. *Figures 7.1* and *7.2* show sample forms that could be used for a prevalence survey. The form shown in *Figure 7.1* should be used to collect data from all patients in the clien group, whereas that shown in *Figure 7.2* is solely for

PRESSURE SORE AUDIT

WARD...............................   DATE...............................

PATIENT	WATERLOW SCORE	PRESSURE SORE PRESENT	SPECIAL MATTRESS/BED

Figure 7-1: Pressure sore audit form

PRESSURE SORE REPORT

| WARD............. | DATE.............. | NAME.............. | Waterlow Score............. |

Was the sore(s) present on admission to ward? Yes/No

Was the patient admitted from?
(please tick)
Home
Community
MHH
GHB
Heartlands
SOH
QEH
City Hospital
Nursing Home
Other – Please state

Date sore first seen.....................

Position of sore:
(please tick)
Sacrum
R Ischial Tuberosity
L Ischial Tuberosity
R Trochanter
L Trochanter
R Heel
L Heel
Other – Please state

Grade of sore:
(see below)

Dressing used:

Seen by Tissue Viability Nurse? Yes/No

Is this the first report on this patient? Yes/No

Progress of sore:
(please tick)
Static
Deteriorating
Not sure
Improving

Any other comments:

Components of Waterlow Score..............
Build/Weight for height..............
Continence..............
Skin type..............
Mobility..............
Sex..............
Age..............
Appetite..............
Tissue Malnutrition..............
Neurological deficit..............
Major surgery..............
Medication..............

Grades of Pressure Sores

1. Redness which blanches under light pressure

2. Redness which does not blanch, blistering or superficial break in skin

3. Break in skin, through to dermis

4. Sore down to subcuticular layer

5. Sore extends to other tissue eg. muscle, tendon, bone

Figure 7–2: Pressure sore audit form for patients with pressure sores

use in patients with pressure sores. A full explanation and training should be given to representatives and/or link nurses from each area such as a ward or a district nursing team. It is also useful to provide written instructions (*Table 7.1*). It should be stressed that the link nurse is responsible for organising the data collection, not for collecting it single-handed.

Table 7.1: Instructions for a prevalence survey

Definition: A point prevalence survey is the measurement of the number of persons with a pressure sore from within a specific patient group measured at a particular point in time

1. The survey will be carried out on ....day/month

2. All patients present in the clinical area at 06.00 hours will be included. This means that all discharges and deaths will be included but not new admissions

3. The information for each patient should be completed by the nurse caring for that patient

4. Figure 7.1 should be completed for all patients in the clinical area

5. Figure 7.2 should only be completed for those patients with pressure sores

6. When all the data have been collected, place in the envelope provided and leave for collection by ....

7. Please contact...................... if you have any problems

Thank you for your assistance

The resources

A whole range of resources needs to be considered. They include standard hospital mattresses, pressure-relieving mattresses and beds, chairs, cushions, equipment for moving patients and wound management products. An inventory will list the items that are available, but their state of repair and suitability also need to be considered. Other issues

MATTRESS-TESTING PROCEDURE
Criteria for Audit

1. Depth of mattress
   All standard mattresses should be 5"/130mm in depth.
   Depth is currently measured at the edge of the mattress using a standard ruler
2. 'Fist test' for foam bottoming out. The bed should be at the lowest height with the mattress cover on:
   a) Link hands to form a fist and place on the mattress
   b) Keep your elbows straight
   c) Lean forward with body weight, and test along the six points of the mattress indicated below

The following should be used as a guide for where to test

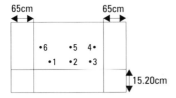

If the foam bottoms out or is nearing bottoming out then the mattress should be withdrawn from service.

3. Condition of foam
   The inner foam should be checked for the following:
   a) Wet or badly stained
   b) Malodour on removing the cover
   If the foam fails on any of these points then the mattress should be withdrawn from service.
4. Condition of the cover
   The mattress cover should be checked for the following:
   a) Damage, split or torn
   b) Excessive staining
   c) Bad fit to mattress
   If the cover fails on point (a) the whole mattress may need to be replaced. If the cover fails on points (b) and (c) then the cover only will need replacing.
5. Dating and numbering
   All new standard mattresses must be numbered and dated. Numbering mattresses helps ensure that mattresses are turned on a regular basis.

They should be numbered from one to four on each corner using a permanent marker, eg. Berol.

Any time a new standard mattress is supplied to the ward it should be dated, again using a permanent marker with a date it first came into use on the ward not the date of delivery to the hospital.

Figure 7-3: Mattress-testing procedure

include maintenance, accessibility and distribution of equipment.

Increasingly, hospitals are recognising that the standard hospital mattress has a limited lifespan. It is important to test all mattresses for grounding, ie. whether the foam has collapsed. *Figure 7.3* illustrates a simple method for testing mattresses. It is unrealistic to expect the nursing staff to test all the mattresses in a clinical area in one day. It is more reasonable to allow 1–2 weeks for collection of the information.

Little information is available for the assessment of armchairs. Dealey *et al* (1991) used three methods for testing armchairs:

Test A: The general condition of the chair — the frame, the covering material and the state of the armrests.

Test B: The condition of the cushion and any obvious indentation.

Test C: The cushion was tested for grounding.

Eden (1995) reported that testing for grounding was more effective than using a visual assessment of cushion indentation. Testing for ground is achieved by pressing the palms of the hands on the chair cushion. If the wooden frame can be felt, then the foam has collapsed.

Baseline knowledge

Identifying the knowledge base of the members of the multidisciplinary team, including that of the pressure sore group, may be a rather more delicate matter. No-one likes to admit ignorance, therefore it is best to ensure anonymity in any survey. Although all disciplines should be included, it should be recognised that the range and level of knowledge may reasonably vary. For example, therapists are likely to have a good understanding of the types of cushions and issues relating to movement, whereas nurses are likely to know more about pressure-relieving mattresses and beds.

Kulkarni and Philbin (1993) conducted a survey of pressure sore awareness among staff in a teaching hospital. The results showed a varying level of knowledge between disciplines, with the medical staff showing less interest in the topic than others. However, 78% of respondents were keen to have further education on pressure sore prevention. It is useful to ask respondents what they consider to be their training needs. It can be of considerable assistance when planning the next stage of policy development, ie. identifying problems and issues.

Identify problems/issues

Once the data have been collected and analysed it is possible to start to identify the relevant issues. The issues that are raised will not necessarily fall neatly under the headings of patients, resources and staff. Many of them will be interlinked. For example, the prevalence survey will have identified the number of patients with pressure sores and their grade and position. An equipment review will have identified any shortfall which may have been relevant to pressure sore development. Dealey *et al* (1991) reported a higher prevalence of sores on the buttocks (38%) than on the sacrum (28%) in a teaching hospital. They also found that only 23% of armchairs were in good condition and that 61% had cushions with grounded foam. They concluded that the poor seating was likely to be a contributing factor in the higher prevalence of pressure sores on the buttocks. Seating was therefore a major issue for this group to resolve.

Another issue is the number of patients at risk of pressure sore development within a clinical area. If a high proportion of patients are found to be at risk then a certain number of 'blanket' strategies can be developed to ensure that patients automatically receive preventive care. Such strategies might involve reviewing the equipment in general use, such as mattresses. The approach is quite different from that in an area where only the occasional patient may be at risk, for example, in a maternity unit.

A number of issues are certain to be raised regarding resources, in addition to those already mentioned. Some equipment may be worn out and require replacement, there may be a shortfall in some areas, there may be inappropriate usage, and there may be no coherent maintenance programme. Some of these issues will apply to dressings, as well as to mattresses, beds and chairs.

The need for more education in some aspects of pressure sore prevention and management is almost certain to be identified. It is helpful to consider the level of knowledge required by all healthcare professionals and the needs of individual disciplines. This will make the task of planning the educational programme much easier.

Develop and implement the policy

The national Clinical Practice Guidelines (Collinson and Hitch, 1995) suggest a number of subheadings which might be used as a basis for developing a policy. They will each be considered in turn.

Patient/carer involvement and education

Any plan of care should involve the patient and/or carers wherever possible. Obviously, this may be limited in the case of a critically ill patient. However, for those at long-term risk full recognition of the patient's knowledge and experience should be given. Patient education is also extremely important. Many patients are able to play an active role in pressure sore prevention. Written information can reinforce the spoken word. A number of trusts have developed their own booklets for patients and carers. The Department of Health has also developed a booklet entitled *Relieving the Pressure — Your Guide to Pressure Sores*. Details of how this may be obtained are given at the end of this chapter.

Risk assessment

The assessment of pressure sore risk should be seen as part of a comprehensive patient assessment. This has been discussed in detail in Chapter 3. The policy should provide guidance on the assessment that is required, including the use of a risk calculator. It should also suggest the frequency of reassessment that is appropriate for the patient population. The national Clinical Practice Guidelines also state that identification of risk should set in motion the development and implementation of an individualised prevention plan.

Classification

It may be helpful to discuss with purchasing authorities their requirements for the minimum data to be collected for patients with pressure damage. One aspect of this will be the grading system to be used. Information regarding the site of the sore and a clinical description may also be required. Certainly, for patient records and for appropriate management, good record keeping is essential. It may also be timely to link the policy to any wound management policy.

Equipment

This section of the policy may take a little time to develop as the pressure sore group may decide to provide some guidance on the selection of equipment for individual patients. This may take the form of a flow chart (Dealey, 1995). It may be necessary to evaluate a number of products over a period of time to identify those suitable for the patient group and when they may best be used. The financial implications must also be remembered. Sometimes a pragmatic approach has to be taken and any strategy may involve the purchase of equipment over a period of time rather than immediate purchase of all the equipment required. Planning the selection of equipment and monitoring its use is a major part of the role of the clinical nurse specialist in tissue viability. Hill (1995) notes that the specialist nurse only rarely has control of the budget.

Education

It is beneficial to include education within the policy as it needs to be a continuous process. Obviously, an educational programme would be part of the launch and implementation process of the new policy. It must be remembered that staff members may change and that regular updating is needed for all members of staff. Including education as part of the policy will also assist in ensuring the support of senior management for the programme.

Continuous quality improvement

This section of the policy includes clinical audit and must be negotiated with local purchasing authorities.

Audit the effect

The final step in establishing a pressure sore prevention policy is the development of a means of auditing the outcomes. This will be discussed in detail in Chapter 8.

Conclusions

Establishing an effective prevention policy can ensure that a coherent approach to pressure sore management is taken across a trust. This is more likely to result in success in reducing the incidence of pressure sores than a haphazard response.

Key points

1.   All trusts and provider units should have a policy for pressure sore prevention

2. A multidisciplinary pressure sore group is needed to establish the policy

3. Baseline information on patients, resources and staff knowledge is required

4. Strategies must take note of the specific problems identified from the baseline data collection.

Useful information

Relieving the Pressure — Your Guide to Pressure Sores, a booklet for patients and carers, can be obtained free of charge by contacting the Health Literature Line on 0800 555 777.

References

Collinson G, Hitch S (1995) *Pressure Sore Prevention and Management: Clinical Practice Guidelines.* Guideline Synopsis. Conference on Clinical Effectiveness from Clinical Guidelines to Cost-Effective Practice, May 3–4, London

Dealey C (1991) The size of the pressure sore problem in a teaching hospital. *J Adv Nurs* **16**: 663–70

Dealey C (1995) Mattresses and beds. *J Wound Care* **4**(9): 409–12

Dealey C, Earwaker T, Eden L (1991) Are your patients sitting comfortably? *J Tissue Viabil* **1**(2): 36–9

Eden L (1995) Testing armchairs. Paper presented at the Tissue Viability Society Spring Conference, 28–29 March

Hill S (1995) The problems that tissue viability nurses have in advising their health authorities on the purchase of pressure relieving equipment. *J Tissue Viabil* **5**(4): 127–9

Kulkarni J, Philbin M (1993) Pressure sore awareness in a university teaching hospital. *J Tissue Viabil* **3**(3): 77–9

Royal College of Physicians (1986) Disability in 1986 and beyond. *J R Coll Physicians Lond* **20**(3): 160–94

Simpson G, Livesley B (1993) *The Prevention and Management of Pressure Sores Within Hospital and Community Settings.* The Research for Ageing Trust, London

Chapter 8

Pressure sore audit

Introduction

A core aim of the NHS is to improve health (NHS Executive, 1993). This can be achieved by improving clinical effectiveness. In order to identify the effectiveness of an intervention the outcome must be measured. An outcome can be defined as a change, either favourable or unfavourable, in the health status of an individual. Outcomes are also sometimes called outcome measures; this is, in part, because they can be measured by the audit process.

Audit has become an important activity in health care and has gradually been extended to most aspects of patient care. The term 'audit' can be defined as 'a searching explanation' (Fowler and Fowler, 1964). Medical audit, especially by means of peer review, has been established for many years. The term 'clinical audit' is relatively new and is meant to encompass all members of the healthcare team. Clinical audit was give a particular impetus by the document *Working for Patients* (Department of Health, 1989).

The following definition has been proposed by the Department of Health (1993a):

'Clinical audit involves systematically looking at the procedures used for diagnosis, care and treatment, examining how associated resources are used and investigating the effect that care has on the outcome and

quality of life for the patient.'

Successful audit has a number of components: audit should be undertaken by the multidisciplinary team; it should be patient-focused; and it should have a culture of continuing evaluation and aim to improve clinical effectiveness. Audit often involves measuring outcomes. Any audit tool that is developed for this purpose should be reliable, valid, responsive, clinically credible and easy to use.

Auditing occurs at different levels. At the ward level, quality issues, such as standards or improving patient records may be considered; at provider unit or directorate level, business plans or policies could be audited. Whereas the purchasing authority might want to look at costs, such as extended stay or opportunity costs relating to pressure sores. At every level, however, the purpose of audit is to improve the quality of care given to patients.

Pressure sores and audit

The development of a pressure sore can be seen as an adverse outcome which impacts on the health status of the individual. The Audit Commission Review (1991) suggested that the incidence of pressure sores could be used as a marker of quality standards within a hospital. Pressure sore incidence has also been described as a key quality indicator (Department of Health, 1993b). As a result there has been much greater interest in the subject of pressure sore prevention. While it is unrealistic to expect to obtain 100% prevention, Waterlow (1988) suggested that 95% of sores could be prevented. *The Health of the Nation* (Department of Health, 1992) proposed a target of 5–10% reduction in the incidence of pressure sores each year.

It is extremely gratifying for those who have long had an interest in pressure sores to find that their managers are now expressing an interest in the management of pressure incidence. However, there are also drawbacks. Policy makers may not have a complete understanding of the aetiology of pressure sores. Unrealistic demands may be made and there have even been rumours of financial penalties for hospitals where patients develop pressure sores. Community nurses are being encouraged to 'inform' on such hospitals. It is extremely important that pressure sore audit is more than just a number-crunching exercise with the temptation to devise league tables. All the elements of pressure sore audit need to be considered.

The elements of pressure sore audit

The patient population

The type of patients being audited should be recognised, as some groups are more vulnerable than others. For example, patients in a maternity hospital are unlikely to be at risk of pressure sore development, whereas many of those in an elderly care unit may be at high risk. Any comparisons should compare like with like. However, it is not always easy to determine what like is. O'Dea (1993) found a pressure sore prevalence of 21.8% among 481 patients in one teaching hospital, whereas (Dealey, 1994), in a survey of another teaching hospital with 405 patients, found it to be 7.9%. Neither survey provided sufficient information about the type of patients cared for in each of these hospitals or the prevention strategies being used. It is much better to monitor the progress within a single hospital than to make spurious comparisons between hospitals.

Prevention policies

Audit should consider what policies have been established for the management and prevention of pressure sores. A number of questions can be asked. Is the policy appropriate? When was it last updated? Does it involve the multidisciplinary team? Is there a copy on each ward? It should also be recognised that a policy has no value if the staff are not aware of its existence. Education programmes are essential to ensuring that staff are equipped to carry out any policy. Audit should include evaluation of the education provided. One hospital showed a reduction in pressure sore prevalence from 13.5% to 5.6% in a year following a training programme using a pressure sore workshop for all staff (NHS Executive, 1993). Another question which might be asked is whether there is a mechanism for patient education. Again, the type of patient must be considered. For example, a more intensive education programme will be needed for patients with spinal injuries who will always be at risk than for those who will only be at risk for a short time.

Equipment

There is increasing use of pressure-relieving equipment. However, it can be misused, used inappropriately or kept in a locked cupboard. Equipment also wears out. An annual audit of all standard mattresses, chairs, trolleys and pressure-relieving equipment will provide useful information about their condition. It should be allied to a maintenance and replacement programme. Consideration should be given to the suitability of equipment for the patient population. For example, the use of water mattresses has largely been discontinued. Although they provided reasonable pressure reduction, they were not suitable for the patient trying to move himself in the bed or trying to rise from sitting on the edge of the bed.

The prevalence of pressure sores

The terms prevalence and incidence are sometimes used interchangeably, but they represent quite different methods of data collection. Prevalence can be defined as:

'The number of persons with a specific disease or condition as a proportion of a given population measured at a specific point in time.'

There are a number of advantages in measuring point prevalence: it provides baseline data about a patient population; it can highlight areas where patients are at particularly high risk; and it can be used over time to measure the effects of prevention policies. However, a prevalence survey identifies all patients with pressure sores and does not necessarily differentiate between those who were admitted with pressure sores and those developing pressure sores in the hospital. It is not as responsive to change as the measurement of incidence.

Measuring incidence

Incidence can be defined as:

'The number of people developing a specific condition as a proportion of the local population measured over a period of time.'

The measurement of incidence is generally a much more costly procedure than measuring prevalence which is usually carried out once a year. Monitoring all patients admitted to a hospital or unit throughout their stay requires regular data collection. While this can be done weekly in longer stay areas, it must be done daily in acute areas. Obviously, computerised methods of data collection are more practical and less time-consuming than manual methods. Once established, however, much more detailed information can be obtained from incidence surveys than from prevalence surveys.

Conclusions

Pressure sore audit can elicit useful information about the quality of care provided by a hospital or unit. It should not just be a number-counting exercise. The precise audit information should be agreed between purchasing authorities and provider units. The type of patients, the effectiveness of the prevention policies, staff education, and the use and maintenance of equipment should all be considered. Improvements in incidence over time in a hospital should be considered more important outcome measures than comparing rates with other hospitals. It is highly unlikely that there are any two identical hospitals in the country with the same numbers of patients at the same degree of risk of developing pressure sores.

Key points

1.   Clinical audit is a suitable method for measuring the effectiveness of healthcare intervention

2.   Pressure sore audit is seen as a method for measuring the quality of care given by a provider unit

3.   Purchasers and providers should agree the data to be collected

4.   Pressure sore audit should consider patient populations, prevention policies and equipment as well as the prevalence and incidence of pressure sores

References

Audit Commission Review (1991) *The Virtue of Patients: Making the Best of Ward Nursing Resources.* The Audit Commission for Local Authorities and the National Health Service in England and Wales, London

Dealey C (1994) Monitoring the pressure sore problem in a teaching hospital. *J Adv Nurs* **20**: 652–9

Department of Health (1989) *Working for Patients*. Department of Health, London

Department of Health (1992) *The Health of the Nation*. HMSO, London

Department of Health (1993a) *Clinical Audit*. Department of Health, London

Department of Health (1993b) *Pressure Sores — A Key Quality Indicator*. Department of Health, London

Fowler HW, Fowler FG (1964) *The Concise Oxford Dictionary of Current English*, 5th edn. Oxford University Press, Oxford

NHS Executive (1993) *The A–Z of Quality*. Department of Health, London: 186

O'Dea K (1993) Prevalence of pressure damage in hospital patients in the UK. *J Wound Care* **2**(4): 221–5

Waterlow J (1988) Prevention is cheaper than cure. *Nurs Times* **84**(25): 69–70

Chapter 9
Conclusions

This chapter seeks to draw together the various threads of the book. A number of facts about pressures sores can be seen as indisputable:

- Pressure sores are a very painful and costly condition

- They occur in those who are either very sick or who suffer from a chronic degenerative condition

- Pressure sores are largely preventable

- The prevention of pressure sores is complex and requires a multidisciplinary approach

There are still a number of areas relating to pressure sores where there are unanswered questions. Further research is required to clarify these issues. Ideally, this should be in the form of randomised controlled trials. However, ethical issues will determine how some of this work may be carried out. For example, if a specific treatment is to be evaluated then suitable patients would normally be randomly allocated to either the 'treatment group' or the 'no treatment group', the latter being the control group. However, in the case of pressure sores it would be unethical not to provide some form of prevention for all of those at risk, including those in the control group. Some form of standard treatment would have to be given, but it is not easy to determine what it should be.

In the 1980s, when many of the modern wound management products were being evaluated, they were often compared with low-adherent dressings as this was considered to be a standard treatment. After a time, this was seen as inappropriate as any product that provides a moist environment and does not adhere to the wound on removal is almost certain to outperform a low-adherent dressing. More emphasis is now given to the need to compare like products.

The recent *Effective Health Care Bulletin* (1995) on pressure sore prevention and treatment suggests that the standard hospital mattress is outperformed by a range of pressure-relieving mattresses and overlays, including pressure- reducing foam mattresses. This type of mattress may be a suitable standard treatment for all but the very high risk patients. However, clear instructions would need to be given for withdrawing patients from treatment in the event of tissue damage.

Cullum (1996) has discussed the need for good quality clinical trials to support healthcare interventions. She proposed a list of features that should be found in a well-constructed clinical trial *(Table 9.1)*. Not every nurse will be involved in carrying out research, but all nurses should be able to critique it and be able to recognise its value, or otherwise, to the advancement of evidence-based health care.

Table 9.1: The features of a well-constructed clinical trial

- Clear inclusion and exclusion criteria

- A clear definition of what is being studied

- A suitable method of randomisation or allocation to the alternative treatments, taking note of the problems of bias

- The use of a recognised current standard treatment in the control group

- The intervention should be the single baseline difference between different patient groups

- Adequate information about withdrawals from the study

- Clear details of adverse events

- Suitable, clinically meaningful outcomes

- Adequate information about the patients

- The sample size should be large enough to provide a meaningful result

- Appropriate statistical analysis

- The results should be published

Based on Cullum (1996)

The areas that require further research are:

Aetiology: The precise mechanism is still uncertain

Risk calculators: Validity and reliability

Manual repositioning: How often is it necessary?

Pressure-relieving equipment: Efficacy and comparability

Other prevention strategies: For example, the role of nutrition

No doubt as some of these questions are answered, others will arise.

Pressure sore prevention is a challenge to the healthcare team, and one that must be met if we are to provide good quality care for our patients. It behoves us to recognise this and take action.

References

Cullum N (1996) Evaluation of treatments for wounds in clinical trials. *J Wound Care* **5**(1): 8–9

Effective Health Care Bulletin (1995) *The Prevention and Treatment of Pressure Sores,* Vol 2(1). Churchill Livingstone and University of York, York

Index